Understanding Liver Cancer:

A Tale of Two Diseases

Understanding Liver Cancer:
A Tale of Two Diseases

Brian I. Carr, MD, FRCP, PhD
Director, Liver Cancer Program
IRCCS de Bellis Medical Center
Castellana Grotte BA
Italy

Published by Springer Healthcare Ltd, 236 Gray's Inn Road, London, WC1X 8HB, UK.

www.springerhealthcare.com

©2014 Springer Healthcare, a part of Springer Science+Business Media.

ISBN 978-1-910315-01-9

Project editor: Tess Salazar
Production manager: Patty Goldstein
Printed in Great Britain by Latimer Trend

Contents

"Everything should be made as simple as possible, but not simpler."
- Albert Einstein

"Truth does not become more true by virtue of the fact that the entire world agrees with it,
nor less so even if the whole world disagrees with it."
- Maimonides, *The Guide for the Perplexed*

"Scientific knowledge is in perpetual evolution; it finds itself changed from one day to the next."
- Jean Piaget

For my children: Ophira and Rajeev, Feridey and Mike
And their children: Rohan, Kunal and Oren

Author biography

Brian I. Carr, MD, FRCP, PhD, was born in Glasgow, Scotland and grew up in London. After graduating from St Mary's Hospital Medical School of the University of London in 1967 he did internships and residencies, including at the Hammersmith Hospital, and a fellowship in Medical Oncology at the Royal Marsden Hospital. Following a PhD in the laboratory of Nobel Laureate Renato Dulbecco at the Imperial Cancer Research Fund (now Cancer Research UK) in London, which he finished in 1977, he moved to the USA, where he has worked since. After a repeat Medical Oncology fellowship at the Wisconsin Clinical Cancer Center in Madison with Paul Carbone and a simultaneous postdoctoral fellowship at the McArdle Laboratory for Cancer Research, he spent 10 years in Los Angeles at the City of Hope Medical Center in Duarte, followed by 20 years at the University of Pittsburgh, Starzl Transplant Institute, as tenured full professor. There he developed a multidisciplinary liver cancer program and co-developed the University of Pittsburgh Liver Cancer Center. He has always worked in both the medical management of liver cancer and the basic science of liver cancer growth stimulatory and inhibitory factors. He has published over 300 papers and this is his third book. He is also the Editor-in-Chief of the *Journal of Gastrointestinal Cancer*.

Abbreviations

AFP	alpha-fetoprotein
ALKP	alkaline phosphatase
CP	Child-Pugh cirrhosis score (A, B, or C)
CT	computed tomography scan
FDA	US Food and Drug Administration
HAI	hepatic artery infusion
HBV	hepatitis B virus
HCC	hepatocellular carcinoma
HCV	hepatitis C virus
LT	liver transplant
MRI	magnetic resonance imaging scan
MWA	microwave ablation
NAFLD	nonalcoholic fatty liver disease
NASH	nonalcoholic steatohepatitis
PVT	portal vein thrombosis
RFA	radiofrequency ablation
TACE	transarterial chemoembolization
VEGF	vascular endothelial growth factor

An extended abbreviation list can be found in Section 6 Addendum (page 50).

Foreword

Until the end of the twentieth century, patients with liver cancer were almost exclusively being taken care of in liver resection and/or transplant centers. As up to 95% of liver cancers arise in patients with liver disease, aggressive treatment (this means liver transplantation) was advocated in order to deal with both conditions, the cancer and the underlying liver disease. Expertise about care and treatment of these patients became thus merely concentrated in liver transplant centers and in oncologic groups working in close collaboration with liver transplant centers.

This situation has been profoundly changed since the recent introduction in clinical practice of several (targeted) medical treatments. As a consequence, hepatocellular cancer moved from its "orphan" disease status (ie, almost no healthcare givers were interested in taking care of these compromised patient groups) to a "desired adoptive" disease status (ie, "everyone" became interested in taking care of these patients). Indeed, such patients are nowadays referred to various medical specialties, including hepatology, gastroenterology, oncology, internal medicine, interventional radiology, radiotherapy, general surgery, liver surgery and (still) liver transplantation. This diverse referral pattern led to a, many times, heterogeneous and even confusing therapeutic algorithm.

Brian Carr's booklet *Understanding Liver Cancer: A Tale of Two Diseases* is, therefore, timely and addressed to the medical profession, with helpful summaries in each chapter. Based on his huge personal experience in this domain of oncology, the author has produced a concise and clear guide to all of the different aspects and problems encountered when dealing with the treatment of patients with liver cancer.

This booklet is of value for every medical caregiver who manages these patients. A better understanding of both diseases is the best guarantee in order to further improve the care of patients with liver cancer. One should also become aware that long-term disease-free outcome is of utmost importance in order to value any liver cancer treatment. In this perspective, carefully selected patients fare best with a liver transplant procedure. It has already been predicted now, based on experiences gathered in the fields of liver surgery, liver transplantation, interventional radiology, radiotherapy and oncology, that inclusion criteria for liver transplantation will be further extended based on both morphologic and biologic tumor behavior. Such extension can, however, only be justified when implementing the sound oncologic principles of neo-adjuvant and adjuvant therapies.

It may be hoped that clear reviews about the subject, such as those expressed in this booklet, may trigger the interest of the medical community to further improve the search towards the optimal treatment of patients with liver cancer.

Professor Jan Lerut
Director UCL Transplant Centre
Director Starzl Abdominal Transplant Unit UCL
Université catholique de Louvain
Brussels
Belgium

Preface

The idea behind this book stems from the apparent complexity of hepatocellular carcinoma (HCC), as its management and prognosis are influenced by two separate yet interacting diseases, namely the underlying liver disease, which is often inflammatory, and the HCC. All textbooks mention this and systematically explore the causes, modifying factors, radiological tests and the many treatment options of both sets of diseases. The aim of this new text is to synthesize these various influences, especially with regard to therapy choices. Also, summaries have been included at intervals throughout the text, which are written with less medical jargon for readers who may not have a medical background, such as patients, families, caregivers and medical non-specialists. Advances in more effective hepatitis therapies, radiological diagnosis, non-surgical (medical) therapies, and therapy combinations have resulted in a flux of new ideas in the last 5 years and this can be expected to continue as various new medical therapies are evaluated in clinical trials, alone or in combination, as well as in combination with surgical therapies. The words cancer/tumor and therapy/treatment are used interchangeably. The basic idea is that this is a tale of two diseases and for patients with HCC, each cannot be considered in isolation any more than treatment options can only be considered in a whole patient context, and by a multidisciplinary team.

Section 1

Introduction to hepatocellular carcinoma: A tale of two diseases

Introduction

Primary liver cancer or hepatocellular carcinoma (HCC) is a tumor of the hepatocyte, the specialized liver epithelial cell that is responsible for most liver function. It is the most common cancer that originates in the liver (primary cancer). By contrast, liver metastases have spread to the liver from cancers arising in other organs and are not further considered here.

Key point
The prognosis and management of HCC are colored and influenced in most patients by the concurrence of two separate but related and interacting liver diseases: hepatitis or cirrhosis from any course on the one hand and HCC on the other hand. It is likely that each influences the other (ie, cirrhosis is a precursor to most HCC and growing HCC can worsen liver function) and the selection of HCC therapy cannot take place without considering the limitations imposed by the concurrent liver disease; thus, it is "a tale of two diseases".

The grading of the degree of HCC differentiation into more or less "hepatocyte-like" features has prognostic significance. On biopsy, the microscopic appearance of poorly differentiated HCCs can look like cancer, while very well-differentiated HCCs may appear more like normal liver cells. Well-differentiated HCCs usually are surrounded by a capsule, but more aggressive HCCs often do not have one and are labeled as "diffuse". HCCs also have a characteristic propensity to invade local blood vessels within the liver (ie, portal vascular invasion or thrombosis [PVT]). A characteristic pattern of reticulin staining is often helpful in pathological diagnosis. The underlying liver is often abnormal, and has varying degrees of necrosis and inflammation, regenerating nodules, and fibrosis, which are the result of chronic injury, usually from hepatitis, and cause cirrhosis. Variant patterns of primary liver tumors, which have quite different behavior, include fibrolamellar HCC of young adults and hepatoblastoma of childhood.

Summary for patients, families, and caregivers
Cancer that starts in the liver is called primary liver cancer, also known as hepatocellular carcinoma or HCC. HCC is closely linked to several other types of inflammatory liver disease. This is because liver diseases can cause HCC and HCC can worsen liver disease. When caring for a patient, healthcare teams must manage the patient's HCC as well as their liver disease. It is a tale of two diseases.
Two types of liver diseases are hepatitis and cirrhosis:
• Hepatitis is an inflammation of the liver. Hepatitis can be caused by a number of factors, including hepatitis viral infections and alcoholism.
• Cirrhosis occurs when scarred or damaged liver tissue from chronic hepatitis replaces healthy liver tissue.
The patient's healthcare team grades and evaluates the patient's HCC and the underlying liver to determine how the cancer might develop and the treatment plan for the patient. Grading is based on analyzing the liver cells under a microscope after a piece of the liver tissue is removed, which is called a needle biopsy.

B. I. Carr, *Understanding Liver Cancer*, DOI: 10.1007/978-1-910315-02-6_1,
© Springer Healthcare 2014

Further reading

1 Carr BI. *Hepatocellular Carcinoma.* 2nd ed. New York, NY: Springer Science+Business Media; 2010.

2 Carr BI. Chapter 92. Tumors of the Liver and Biliary Tree. In: Longo DL, Fauci AS, Kasper DL, et al, eds. *Harrison's Principles of Internal Medicine.* 18th edition. New York, NY: The McGraw-Hill Companies, Inc; 2012:777-785.

3 Carr BI. Chapter 111. Tumors of the Liver and Biliary Tree. In: Longo DL, Fauci AS, Kasper DL, et al, eds. *Harrison's Principles of Internal Medicine.* 19th edition. New York, NY: The McGraw-Hill Companies, Inc; 2014: in press.

Incidence and geography

HCC is the sixth most common cancer worldwide and the third most common cause of death from cancer; the reason for this discrepancy is due to the fact that a high proportion of patients die from this disease (overall ratio of mortality to incidence is about 0.9). There are about 750,000 new global cases annually; it is the fifth most common cancer in males and the seventh most common in females. There is a male predominance in incidence, varying from 9:1 male: female to 2:1 male: female cases, depending on the country, except in low-cirrhosis Western countries where the ratio approaches 1:1 (Figure 1). Possible contributors to the high male incidence include tobacco smoking and alcohol consumption, which are known contributory factors to risk of HCC development.

Most HCC cases worldwide occur in developing countries (Figure 1). The world's highest incidence rates are found in Eastern Asia, followed by Southeast Asia then Central Africa. Southern

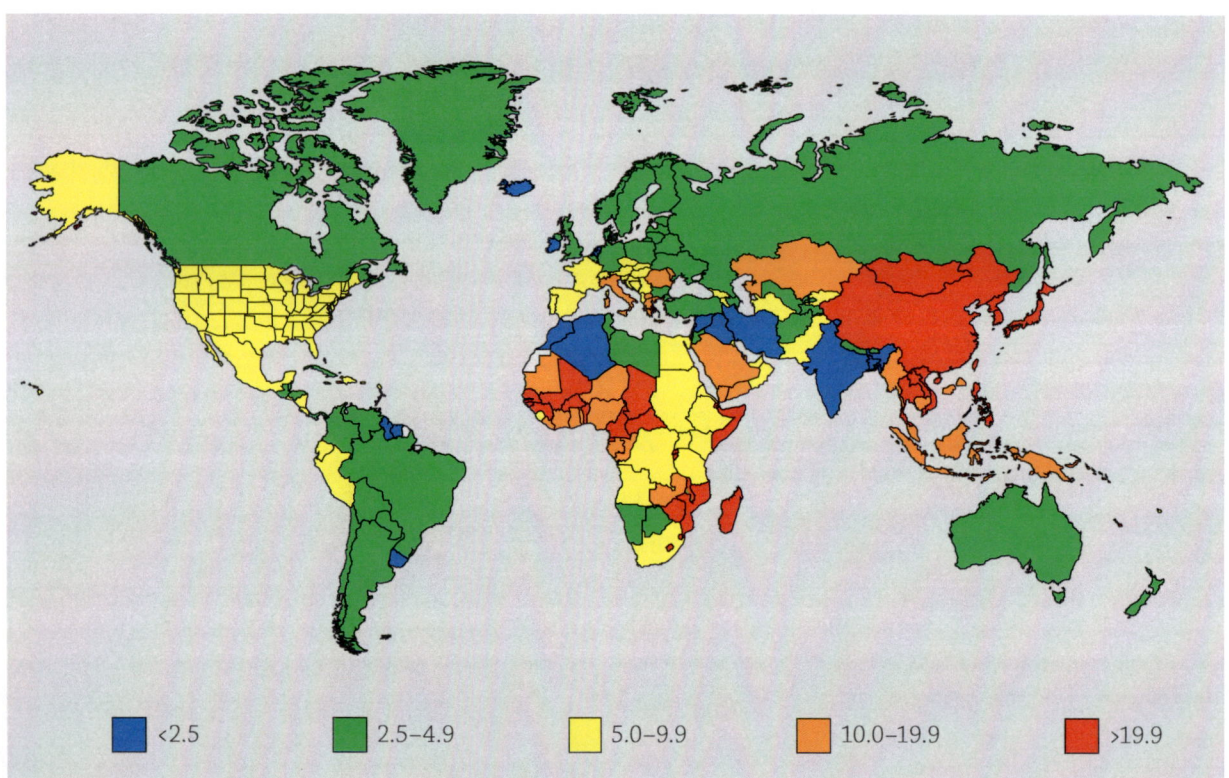

Figure 1 Age-standardized incidence rates of primary liver cancer worldwide, 2002. Reproduced with permission from © GLOBOCAN, 2014; International Agency for Research on Cancer. GLOBOCAN 2012: Estimated Cancer Incidence Mortality and Prevalence Worldwide in 2012. Liver. globocan.iarc.fr/Pages/fact_sheets_cancer.aspx. Accessed January 10, 2014; © Elsevier Limited, 2014; Nordenstedt H, White DL, El-Serag HB. The changing pattern of epidemiology in hepatocellular carcinoma. *Dig Liver Dis.* 2010;42 Suppl 3:S206-S214.

Europe has moderately high rates, as does Central America and Polynesia. Low rates occur in Western Europe, the USA, and South America, with the lowest being in Northern Europe, Australia/New Zealand, and South Central Asia (Figure 2). The large global variation is thought to be due to differences in exposure to causative factors, such as hepatitis virus or carcinogen contamination of foodstuffs, but not to ethnicity. Supporting this, studies of migrant populations, such as Japanese or Jews living in various locales, show changes in HCC incidence in the same ethnic group, but living in different locations.

In the USA, HCC is the fifth most common cancer in men after lung, prostate, colon, and pancreas cancers. It was recently estimated that there were approximately 31,000 new annual cases of HCC in the USA in 2013 (23,000 male, 8000 female). In the last 30 years there has been a steady increase in incidence of HCC in the USA, especially among Hispanics, Blacks, and White middle-age people, likely attributable to the hepatitis C (HCV) epidemic, as well as the rising levels of obesity and diabetes. There are clear differences in incidence within the USA population (Table 1) but the differences between males and females in both incidence and mortality are preserved. In Japan, the incidence is thought to have peaked due to the increased screening of blood in blood banks for hepatitis viruses, while in Taiwan and China it is set to decrease due to widespread hepatitis B (HBV) neonatal vaccination.

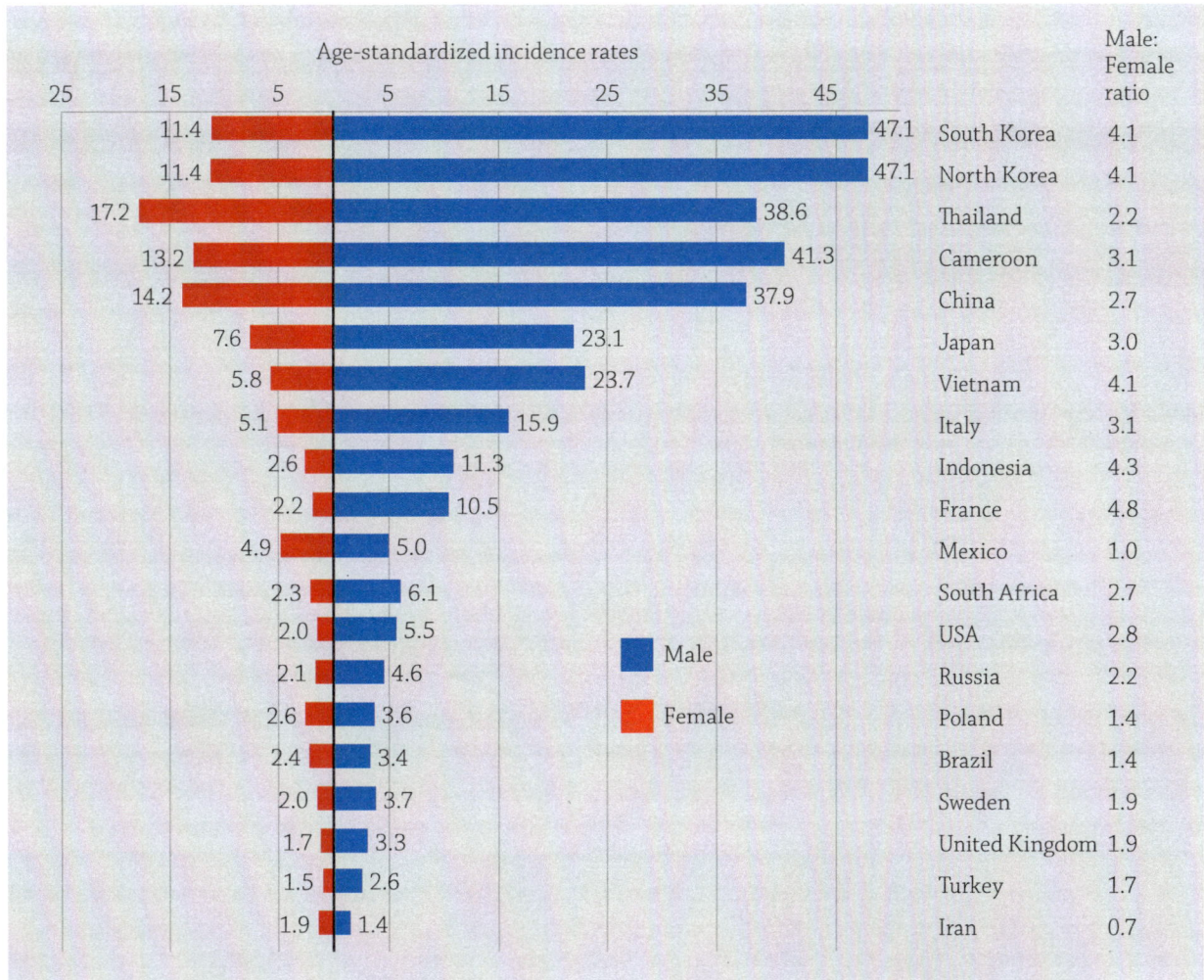

Figure 2 Age-standardized incidence rates of primary liver cancer, per 100,000 population at risk.
Reproduced with permission from © GLOBOCAN, 2014; International Agency for Research on Cancer. GLOBOCAN 2012: Estimated Cancer Incidence Mortality and Prevalence Worldwide in 2012. Liver. globocan.iarc.fr/Pages/fact_sheets_cancer. aspx. Accessed January 10, 2014; © Elsevier Limited, 2014; Nordenstedt H, White DL, El-Serag HB. The changing pattern of epidemiology in hepatocellular carcinoma. *Dig Liver Dis*. 2010;42 Suppl 3:S206-S214.

	White	African American	Asian American	American Indian and Alaskan	Hispanic/ Latino
Incidence, all cancers					
Male	543	619	328	423	419
Female	424	397	286	360	333
Incidence, liver and bile duct cancers					
Male	**9.1**	**15**	**21.6**	**16**	**17.5**
Female	**3.1**	**4.2**	**8.1**	**7.6**	**6.6**
Mortality, all cancers					
Male	217	288	133	185	146
Female	151	175	93	136	101
Mortality, liver and bile duct cancers					
Male	**7.4**	**12**	**14.5**	**13**	**12**
Female	**3.1**	**4**	**6.1**	**6**	**5**

Table 1 Incidence and death rate per 100,000, United States, 2005–2009. Population by site, race, and ethnicity. Per 100,000 population, age adjusted to the 2000 US standard population. Adapted with permission from © John Wiley and Sons, 2014; Siegel R, Naishadham D, Jemal A. Cancer Statistics, 2013. *CA Cancer J Clin*. 2013;63:11-30.

The cause of the gender discrepancy in HCC arising from cirrhosis (>80% of HCC cases) is unclear for viral causes. However, for chemical causes, such as aflatoxin B_1 contamination of foods, animal studies have shown that male rodent livers are better able to metabolize the carcinogen to its DNA reactive and thus carcinogenic form.

Summary for patients, families, and caregivers

Globally, HCC is the sixth most common type of cancer and the third most common cause of death from cancer. The number of new HCC cases varies from country to country. Asian and sub-Saharan African countries have more new cases of HCC than Western countries. This difference is probably due to how each population is exposed to different risk factors. Examples of these risk factors include having hepatitis or eating food that is contaminated by fungal toxins. Generally, men have a higher rate of HCC than women. This may be due increased tobacco smoking and alcohol consumption. Both smoking and drinking are risk factors for developing HCC.

Further reading

1   Siegel R, Naishadham D, Jemal A. Cancer Statistics, 2013. *CA Cancer J Clin*. 2013;63:11-30.
2   International Agency for Research on Cancer. GLOBOCAN 2012: Estimated Cancer Incidence Mortality and Prevalence Worldwide in 2012. Liver. globocan.iarc.fr/Pages/fact_sheets_ cancer.aspx. Accessed January 10, 2014.
3   Couto OF, Dvorchik I, Carr BI. Causes of death in patients with unresectable hepatocellular carcinoma. *Dig Dis Sci*. 2007;52:3285-3289.
4   Nordenstedt H, White DL, El-Serag HB. The changing pattern of epidemiology in hepatocellular carcinoma. *Dig Liver Dis*. 2010;42 Suppl 3:S206-S214.

Causes of hepatocellular carcinoma

Risk factors for developing HCC in patients with cirrhosis include older age, male gender, and severity of compensated cirrhosis, independent of etiology or cause of the cirrhosis (most commonly from hepatitis B virus [HBV], hepatitis C virus [HCV] or alcoholism). Mixed infection with HBV and HCV,

HCV and HIV, or HBV plus alcohol greatly increase the HCC risk as well; common factors associated with an increased risk for developing HCC are:

- Cirrhosis from any cause
- HBV or HCV chronic infection
- Alcohol chronic consumption
- NASH/NAFLD (nonalcoholic steatohepatitis, typically from obesity)
- Aflatoxin B_1 or other mycotoxin contaminated foods

Less common factors associated with an increased risk for developing HCC are:

- Primary biliary cirrhosis
- Hemochromatosis (increased iron)
- α_1 Antitrypsin deficiency
- Glycogen storage diseases (rare metabolic diseases)
- Citrullinemia (rare metabolic disease)
- Porphyria cutanea tarda (rare metabolic disease)
- Hereditary tyrosinemia (rare metabolic disease)
- Tyrosinemia type I (rare metabolic disease)
- Wilson's disease (increased copper)
- Autoimmune hepatitis
- Alagille syndrome of infants

Patients with any of the diseases that predispose them to HCC can be exposed to a variety of additional factors that increase their risk for HCC, including diet, alcohol and possibly obesity.

In addition, a wide range of factors in the human diet can cause HCC in experimental animals, as well as many industrial compounds. Several dietary factors, such as coffee and flavonoids, are also thought to be protective against cancer development (carcinogenesis) (Table 2).

Cirrhosis from any cause predisposes patients to a higher risk of developing HCC. Cirrhosis can typically take 10–15 years to develop after hepatitis viral infection, and HCC typically develops after an additional 10 years or more of chronic infection; cirrhosis is thus a pre-malignant disease. Many patients may die of liver failure from their cirrhosis without developing HCC. Conversely, many patients with cirrhosis can receive curative liver transplants without developing HCC. Cirrhosis occurs in about 10–15% of alcoholics, of whom about 15–20% develop HCC at a rate of 3–4% per annum. Alcohol is not a direct carcinogen, but HCC likely develops as a consequence of alcohol-induced oxidative stress (reactive oxygen species), which then affects downstream cellular lipids, proteins, DNA, and cell signaling pathways. Reactive oxygen species are also thought to be important in iron and copper accumulation disorders as well as in nonalcoholic steatohepatitis (NASH), resulting from fatty liver disease.

The emerging obesity epidemic is associated with NASH, which requires liver biopsy for diagnosis and may also lead to a symptomless form of cirrhosis. NASH is distinct from the usually harmless fatty liver by being associated with liver inflammation. Nonalcoholic fatty liver disease (NAFLD) may or may not be associated with NASH. NAFLD is associated with metabolic syndrome and diabetes mellitus type 2, which in turn can be associated with HCC.

The major cause of HCC in Asia (where HCC is globally most prevalent) and sub-Saharan Africa is chronic HBV. There are over 300 million HBV carriers worldwide who may develop HCC with or without the development of the intermediate step of cirrhosis, unlike HCV in Western countries, where cirrhosis is an intermediate step. The conversion rate for chronic HBV carriers to HCC is thought to be approximately 2–3% per annum. HBV is a DNA-binding virus and may directly influence gene function. The incidence of HCC is lower in alcoholic cirrhosis, NASH and hereditary hemochromatosis. In China, Southeast Asia, and sub-Saharan Africa, aflatoxin B_1 is the most potent naturally occurring liver chemical carcinogen known (a group 1 carcinogen) and is a fungal product that contaminates stored rice, peanuts, ground nuts, and maize, and is an important cause of HCC. The carcinogen is produced by the carcinogenic fungi *Aspergillus flavus* and *Aspergillus parasiticus*. Concomitant HBV plus alcohol as well as HBV plus aflatoxin B_1 exposure are thought to substantially increase the HCC risk; less is known of aflatoxin B_1 combinations with HCV.

A	Complete carcinogens
1	*Aflatoxins – fungal contamination of stored rice and grains; Ochratoxin A
2	Nitrosamines – fried bacon, cured meats
3	Hydrazines – found in edible mushrooms (false morel)
4	Safrole – found in sassafras plant and black pepper. Oil of sassafras in "natural" sarsaparilla root beer is 75% safrole
5	Pyrrolizidine alkaloids – found in herbs, herbal teas, and occasionally in honey (eg, senkirkine [coltsfoot], symphyline [comfrey])
6	Estrogens – from wheat germ, unpolished rice, forage crops
7	Bracken fern carcinogen
8	Methylazoxymethanol or cycasin (cycad plants)
9	Carrageenan – from red seaweeds
10	Tannins – from tea, wine, and plants
11	Ethyl carbamate in some wines, beers
B	Carcinogens from food containing molds and bacteria
1	Aflatoxins (*Aspergillus*)
2	Sterigmatocystin (*Aspergillus versicolor*)
3	Microcystins – from Cyanobacteria in drinking water in China
C	Tumor antagonists
1	Selenium
2	Coffee
3	Antioxidants
4	Phytochemicals, including polyphenols (curcumin from turmeric; resveratrol from red wine)
5	Vitamins A, K, and D. Vitamin A analog (polyprenoic acid, an acyclic retinoid)
6	Flavonols
7	Fish consumption
8	Vitamin K_2 or with polyprenoic acid (an acyclic retinoid)

Table 2 Compounds of natural origin in the human diet that are carcinogenic to experimental animals.
*Only aflatoxins have strong epidemiologic evidence of association with human HCC. Reproduced with permission from © John Wiley and Sons, 2014; Carr BI. Chemical carcinogens and inhibitors of carcinogenesis in the human diet. *Cancer.* 1985;55:218-224.

The major risk factor for developing HCC in Japan, Western Europe, and the USA is by contracting HCV-mediated cirrhosis, mainly from transfusion with contaminated blood or use of contaminated syringes or needles through medical or recreational drug use. The mechanism of HCV-mediated carcinogenesis is complex and it does not bind to DNA like HBV. It is thought that the risk for HCC development in HCV-based cirrhosis is approximately 3–5% per year. HCV seems to relate to HCC mainly via the development of cirrhosis and the risk seems proportional to the severity and duration of the HCV-induced hepatic inflammation and fibrosis that are part of the resulting cirrhosis. Studies involving outbreaks of HCV from contaminated blood transfusions have indicated that it takes decades to develop HCC. However, now that donors and their blood in blood banks can be screened for HCV, it is thought that HCV infections will sharply decrease over the next 30 years. Evidence of this trend is already clearly available in Japan.

Given that the severity of cirrhosis is both an HCC risk factor for patients with HCV and also limits the liver tolerance to surgery or chemotherapy, it is necessary to know the severity of a patient's cirrhosis as graded by the Child-Pugh (CP) score (Table 3). The CP score is categorized as:

- CP A: normal liver function
- CP B: intermediate liver dysfunction
- CP C: severe liver dysfunction

In CP C, the only treatment that the liver can tolerate is complete replacement by transplantation. The 1-year survival with a CP C score, with or without HCC, is only 45% on average, without liver

A Child-Pugh score for cirrhosis grade

Factor	1 point	2 points	3 points
Total bilirubin (μmol/L)	<35	35–50	>50
Serum albumin (g/L)	>35	28–35	<28
PT INR	<1.7	1.71–2.30	>2.30
Ascites	none	mild	moderate/severe
Encephalopathy	none	mild	severe
Scores	**Class A**	**Class B**	**Class C**
	5–6 points	7–9 points	10–15 points
	100% 1-year survival	80% 1-year survival	45% 1-year survival

B Some staging systems for hepatocellular carcinoma

CLIP classification*

	Variables	0 points	1 point	2 points
i	Tumor number	Single	Multiple	–
	Hepatic replacement by tumor	<50%	<50%	>50%
ii	Child-Pugh score	A	B	C
iii	α Fetoprotein level (ng/mL)	<400	≥400	–
iv	Portal vein thrombosis (CT)	No	Yes	–

Okuda classification†

Tumor extent‡		Ascites		Albumin (g/L)		Bilirubin (mg/dL)	
≥50%	<50	+	–	≤3	>3	≥3	<3
(+)	(–)	(+)	(–)	(+)	(–)	(+)	(–)

Table 3 Staging of cirrhosis and hepatocellular carcinoma. A, Child-Pugh score for cirrhosis grade; **B,** staging systems for hepatocellular carcinoma. *CLIP stages (score = sum of points): CLIP 0, 0 points; CLIP 1, 1 point; CLIP 2, 2 points; CLIP 3, 3 points; †Okuda stages: stage 1, all (–); stage 2, 1 or 2 (+); stage 3, 3 or 4 (+); ‡Extent of liver occupied by tumor. CLIP, Cancer of the Liver Italian Program; CT, computed tomography scan; PT INR, prothrombin time international normalized ratio.

transplantation. Thus, to make treatment decisions and survival estimations, both the patient's tumor characteristics and the severity of liver damage need to be taken into account (see page 25). In this respect, HCC differs from most other cancers, such as breast or colon cancer, for which only tumor factors are the primary treatment and prognostic concern.

Macroenvironmental factors appear to influence the incidence and prognosis of HCC. It is a male dominant disease in its incidence, and males with HCC also tend to have more aggressive disease and shorter survival rates than females. This has given rise to past attempts to use hormonal therapies, such as tamoxifen (a breast cancer drug). A large number of trials led to a meta-analysis showing tamoxifen actually had little impact on survival. A similar negative result was obtained for anti-androgen therapy (ie, anandrone plus/minus goserelin). Age is also an important macroenvironmental risk factor. As with most other cancers, HCC has a peak incidence in the 60-year age group. However, very old people tend to have slower growing tumors with a better prognosis, while young people (<35 years) tend to have a quite aggressive tumor biology.

Summary for patients, families, and caregivers

The most common risk factors for developing HCC include: scarring of the liver (cirrhosis), chronic hepatitis B or C viral infection, heavy drinking, fatty liver disease caused by obesity, and eating foods that have been contaminated by cancer-causing fungal toxins.

Continues over

Summary for patients, families, and caregivers (continued)

Cirrhosis is a leading cause of HCC. Cirrhosis is often caused by a hepatitis C infection or alcoholism. Cirrhosis happens when the liver cells become damaged and scar tissue replaces healthy tissue. This stops the liver from working properly. Cirrhosis-associated inflammation increases the risk of developing HCC. The healthcare team must know how severe a patient's cirrhosis is to determine if they can tolerate surgery or chemotherapy to treat their HCC. However, liver transplantation can be safely performed in presence of any degree of cirrhosis severity.

The leading cause of HCC in Asia and sub-Saharan Africa is hepatitis B infection. Patients have a higher risk for developing HCC if they have hepatitis B infection and are alcoholics or have hepatitis B infection and are exposed to fungal toxins.

The leading cause of HCC in Japan, Western Europe, and the USA is cirrhosis that is caused by hepatitis C. People can get hepatitis C through contaminated blood transfusions, syringes, needles, or drug abuse.

Further reading

1 Fattovich G, Stroffolini T, Zagni I, Donato F. Hepatocellular carcinoma in cirrhosis: incidence and risk factors. *Gastroenterology*. 2004;127(5 Suppl 1):S35-S50.

2 Carr BI. Chemical carcinogens and inhibitors of carcinogenesis in the human diet. *Cancer*. 1985;55:218-224.

3 Carr BI. Chapter 92. Tumors of the Liver and Biliary Tree. In: Longo DL, Fauci AS, Kasper DL, et al, eds. *Harrison's Principles of Internal Medicine*. 18th edition. New York, NY: The McGraw-Hill Companies, Inc; 2012.

4 Liu Y, Wu F. Global burden of aflatoxin-induced hepatocellular carcinoma: A risk assessment. *Environ Health Perspect*. 2010;118:818-824.

5 Zamora-Ros R, Fedirko V, Trichopoulou A, et al. Dietary flavonoid, lignan and antioxidant capacity and risk of hepatocellular carcinoma in the European prospective investigation into cancer and nutrition study. *Int J Cancer*. 2013;133:2429-2443.

6 Fedirko V, Trichopolou A, Bamia C, et al. Consumption of fish and meats and risk of hepatocellular carcinoma: the European Prospective Investigation into Cancer and Nutrition (EPIC). *Ann Oncol*. 2013;24:2166-2173.

7 Welzel TM, Graubard BI, Quraishi S, et al. Population-attributable fractions of risk factors for hepatocellular carcinoma in the United States. *Am J Gastroenterol*. 2013;108:1314-1321.

8 Buch SC, Kondragunta V, Branch RA, Carr BI. Gender-based outcomes differences in unresectable hepatocellular carcinoma. *Hepatol Int*. 2008;2:95-101.

9 Carr BI, Pancoska P, Branch RA. HCC in older patients. *Dig Dis Sci*. 2010;55:3584-3590.

Prevention

Prevention and early detection can critically affect outcomes for any disease, especially cancer. Prevention can only be rationally planned when the causes or predisposing factors for a disease are known or determined to be highly likely. As previously mentioned, the most common causes of HCC are chronic HBV infection, chronic HCV infection-associated cirrhosis, mycotoxin (ie, aflatoxin B_1) contamination of foodstuffs, such as peanuts and maize, chronic alcohol-associated cirrhosis, and obesity-associated fatty liver. These are all preventable risk factors.

Primary prevention

Destroying aflatoxin B_1-contaminated, spoiled foodstuffs is simple in theory, but can result in a major financial burden to farmers in impoverished regions in rural China or Africa where it is most common. Prevention of the *Aspergillus* mold from growing in the first place, by storing grains, such as peanuts in refrigerated silos, is likely the most effective preventive measure in these areas, but requires capital outlay for refrigeration in these farming communities.

The near-universal neonatal vaccination against HBV is already showing dramatic decreases in both HBV and the resulting HCC in children and adolescents in those areas with a high incidence of HBV. This approach is likely to cause a huge decrease in Asian HCC in the coming decades.

The elimination of HCV-contaminated blood in blood banks in Europe and Asia is expected to contribute to a major decrease in HCV infection, although recreational drug abuse remains a problem.

Secondary prevention

Once HBV infection has taken place, viral treatment strategies are needed and have become increasingly effective in recent years in decreasing the blood-viral load (sustained virological response). It is expected that this will interfere with the development of cirrhosis and minimize the development of HCC. Although the data are preliminary, some suggestive evidence has been published from meta-analyses of the effectiveness of HBV therapy. The treatment of chronic HCV infection has so far been less effective than that for HBV, but new and more potent therapies have been recently announced and have received US Food and Drug Administration (FDA) approval. Their treatment effects on subsequent HCC development are not yet known, but sustained virological responses in patients with HCV following treatment with these new antiviral therapies may translate into a lower incidence of subsequent HCC development. For both patients with chronic HBV and chronic HCV, a treatment-induced sustained virological response has been found in several studies to reduce the HCC incidence rate by >50%. It remains to be determined if this will be true of patients with HCV who also have cirrhosis.

Since alcohol consumption is a lifestyle choice and a contributor to HCC development, it would seem that alcohol counseling might be effective in either alcohol consumers or for alcohol consumers who are also HBV or HCV carriers, but the effects of an intervention are likely to be greater when undertaken at younger age or at earlier phases of the hepatitis.

Summary for patients, families, and caregivers

Many risk factors for developing HCC can be prevented. There are two methods of prevention: primary and secondary prevention.

- Primary prevention is a method for reducing the chance of developing HCC before it begins. For example, primary prevention includes: destroying contaminated food, vaccinating women (and thus protecting their unborn babies) against hepatitis B, and screening blood at blood banks for hepatitis C. Currently, the most important is vaccinating newborns (neonates) against hepatitis B.
- Secondary prevention means the patient has risk factors, and their healthcare team is trying to prevent HCC from developing. Examples of secondary prevention include: treating patients who have chronic hepatitis B or C infections with antiviral therapy and reducing alcohol consumption. Note: hepatitis A infections do not cause HCC development.

Further reading

1   Ferenci P, Fried M, Labrecque D, et al; World Gastroenterology Organisation Guidelines and Publications Committee. World Gastroenterology Organisation Guideline. Hepatocellular carcinoma (HCC): a global perspective. *J Gastrointestin Liver Dis*. 2010;19:311-317.

2   Singh S, Singh PP, Roberts LR, Sanchez W. Chemopreventive strategies in hepatocellular carcinoma. *Nat Rev Gastroenterol Hepatol*. 2014;11:45-54.

3   Chang MH. Prevention of hepatitis B virus infection and liver cancer. *Recent Results Cancer Res*. 2014;193:75-95.

4   Turati F, Trichopoulos D, Polesel J, et al. Mediterranean diet and hepatocellular carcinoma. *J Hepatol*. 2014;60:606-611. Nov 14. [Epub ahead of print].

5   Thiele M, Gluud LL, Dahl EK, Krag A. Antiviral therapy for prevention of hepatocellular carcinoma and mortality in chronic hepatitis B: systematic review and meta-analysis. *BMJ Open.* 2013;3:1.

6   Morgan RL, Baack B, Smith BD, Yartel A, Pitasi M, Falck-Ytter Y. Eradication of hepatitis C virus infection and the development of hepatocellular carcinoma: a meta-analysis of observational studies. *Ann Intern Med.* 2013;158:329-337.

7   Hosaka T, Suzuki F, Kobayashi M, et al. Long-term entecavir treatment reduces hepatocellular carcinoma incidence in patients with hepatitis B virus infection. *Hepatology.* 2013;58:98-107.

Surveillance screening

As HCC is one of the few human cancers with mostly known causes (particularly from chronic HBV or HCV infection or alcoholism), surveillance or screening is useful in those patients who are known to be at risk, in order to diagnose the disease at an earlier and potentially curable stage.

There are two aims of surveillance screening:

1. To diagnose HCC at early stages of its growth and at a small size, when curative therapies are more feasible and more effective. These therapies include resection, radiofrequency ablation (RFA) and transplantation. Several studies have shown the benefits of this for HBV carriers, but less so for HCV carriers who have developed cirrhosis.

2. To begin these therapies earlier in the tumor growth trajectory, with the assumption that they will result in longer survival rates for patients. Until recently, the evidence for this aim was not available. However, recent preliminary evidence strongly suggests that there may also be a survival benefit, especially amongst HBV carriers. Performing randomized studies are difficult for screening, as most patients with chronic hepatitis will not willingly agree to not be screened, and thus to not have their tumor diagnosed at earlier and thus treatable stages.

Consensus screening recommendations advise that abdominal ultrasound examinations should be performed every 6–12 months for patients with diseases that put them at risk for developing HCC; however, a recent study showed there was no survival difference between 6- and 12-monthly screenings. Screening and surveillance guidance based on tumor size is explained in Table 4.

There has been much debate as to whether screening should also include the blood alpha-fetoprotein (AFP) test. In the absence of ultrasound availability in poor or rural areas of the third world, there is consensus that AFP tests should be used. In this author's view, AFP is inexpensive and easy to measure in routine clinical laboratories and thus should be included with ultrasound testing. Elevated levels can also occur in association with hepatitis without HCC, but levels >400 ng/ml are accepted as suspicious for presence of HCC. Around 50% of patients with HCC do not have elevations of AFP levels, so normal values do not exclude the presence of HCC. Whereas AFP can be increased in hepatitis as well as HCC, the two newer markers (both FDA-approved for clinical use in diagnosis) AFP-L3 and des-gamma carboxy prothrombin are HCC-specific; in Japan, the consensus is to measure all three markers (there is a combination kit) in patients at risk for developing HCC.

Summary for patients, families, and caregivers

Screening for HCC is possible because it has several known risk factors. The earlier the cancer is detected by screening, the sooner it can be treated. Furthermore, preliminary evidence shows that patients who are treated early have longer survival rates.

Screening for HCC involves an abdominal ultrasound scan. This ultrasound scan can determine if there is a tumor, its potential size, and possibly its growth after repeated scans. Abdominal ultrasound scans should be performed every 6–12 months for patients at risk for developing HCC. Screening can also include a cheap blood test that is called an alpha-fetoprotein (AFP) test.

1	≤1 cm diameter nodule	Repeat scan every 3–6 months for 2 years, if stable
		If growing, evaluate with contrast CT or MRI, looking for lesion hypervascularity on the arterial phase followed by venous or delayed phase washout. If typical, treat as HCC. If atypical, biopsy needed
2	1–2 cm diameter nodule	Evaluate as per growing lesion above
3	>2 cm diameter lesion	CT or MRI as above plus serum AFP measurement. If AFP >200 ng/ml, high probability of HCC

Table 4 Evaluation of a suspicious liver nodule found on surveillance ultrasound scan in patients with cirrhosis or chronic hepatitis B infection. AFP, alpha-fetoprotein; CT, computed tomography scan; HCC, hepatocellular carcinoma; MRI, magnetic resonance imaging scan.

Further reading

1   Yuen MF, Cheng CC, Lauder IJ, Lam SK, Ooi CG, Lai CL. Early detection of hepatocellular carcinoma increases the chance of treatment: Hong Kong experience. *Hepatology*. 2000;31:330-335.

2   Sangiovanni A, Colombo M. Surveillance for hepatocellular carcinoma: a standard of care, not a clinical option. *Hepatology*. 2011;54:1898-1900.

3   Singal AG, Nehra M, Adams-Huet B, et al. Detection of hepatocellular carcinoma at advanced stages among patients in the HALT-C trial: where did surveillance fail? *Am J Gastroenterol*. 2013;108:425-432.

Biology of human hepatocellular carcinoma

Important principles of the biology of HCC will be presented in this section, which may help when evaluating an individual patient and determining a management approach.

Primary drug resistance

For most other cancers that have been studied, after a given number of chemotherapy treatments, the tumors can adapt and become resistant to the cell-killing effects of the chemotherapy. This is called secondary or acquired resistance, and is similar to the resistance seen in bacteria after exposure to antibiotics or in insects to insecticides. HCC is different in that it has primary resistance to a huge array of toxins and most chemotherapeutics. Work done decades ago showed that cells that develop in a chronic toxic/carcinogenic milieu acquire a pan-drug resistance phenotype when they become cancers. This is called primary resistance. Thus, trying to overcome this resistance with high doses of chemotherapeutic agents, especially in the presence of chronic liver damage, is often futile at best and dangerous for the liver at worst. Perhaps this is why such a large number of chemotherapy clinical trials failed to produce any meaningful survival advantage for patients with HCC, and could be usually only done in selected patients.

Vascular characteristics

There are two different vascular characteristics of HCC. First, it is one of the most vascular of tumors, and HCC has distinctive features on computed tomography (CT) and magnetic resonance imaging (MRI) scans. Unlike other organs, most of the liver's oxygenated blood, approximately 95%, comes from the portal vein and not from a feeding artery. In contrast, around 80% of oxygenated blood for HCCs comes from arterial outgrowths from hepatic arterial branches. This was noted 30 years ago in Japan to offer a potential means for delivering drugs/chemotherapy moderately selectively to the tumor by injecting them into the hepatic artery and thus minimizing the exposure of the underlying diseased liver to the drug toxicities; however, the liver is only partially protected because in cirrhosis there is hepatic arterial blood shunting and direct intrahepatic arteriovenous connections open up.

A second characteristic of HCC is the propensity of HCC cells to invade the portal vein and grow in its lumen. When the portal vein is occluded, a characteristic enlargement and vascular enhancement is seen on CT. This is called macrovascular venous invasion (PVT) as shown in Figure 3, in contrast to microvascular venous invasion that is only seen on biopsy or in pathology liver specimens. Because the tumor cells are now in a vein, they can/do get carried by the blood stream around the circulation, with the possibility of forming distant metastases. Macrovascular invasion very often results in post-liver transplant recurrences and is thus considered a contraindication to this surgery. Microvascular invasion does not seem to carry such a great risk. The reasons are unclear, as the cells are also within the venous lumen (inside the vein). Main branch PVT is considered to be a contraindication to transarterial chemoembolization (TACE)/chemoembolization, as disease has blocked the portal vein and the TACE/chemoembolization therapy blocks the artery, so the affected liver lobe loses its blood supply and can be severely damaged. Often, if only one of the two major portal vein branches is blocked by the tumor (branch PVT), then the therapy can still be safely given to the other side of the liver.

Hepatocellular carcinoma growth rates

HCCs have been reported to have a wide range of doubling times (growth rates) from one month to a year. Without repeated scans over several months or more, it is impossible to calculate the tumor growth rate of HCC in an individual patient. A newly diagnosed patient could have had a slow growing 5 cm HCC for 3 years (Figure 4, red line); another patient with the same size tumor on the first clinic visit might have had only a 2 cm tumor 6 months ago and will thus have an aggressively behaving tumor (Figure 4, blue line). On that first visit without the knowledge of prior scans, it would have been impossible to know the growth rate of the tumor. Thus, patients are quite heterogeneous with respect to their tumor biology and characteristics.

Size alone may not be so important, as many large HCCs with >8 cm diameter can arise in noncirrhotic liver and are thus quite resectable. Fast growing tumors are often associated with several "satellite" lesions likely because they "seed" the surrounding liver. However, there is another mechanism for multifocality, as the presence of PVT is also a means of tumor spread within the liver (more common than distant metastases). This has significance for resection surgery, where up to 40% of patients have recurrence within 5 years after supposedly curative surgery. Such recurrences are observed to be "early" within a few months or "late" after a year or more, which have different causes. Early recurrence tends to be near the resection site and close to where the removed tumor was located; it is thought to be direct tumor extension from cells that could not have been seen at surgery or on the preresection scan. The late recurrences are often in other parts of the liver and may be new primary HCCs. In cirrhosis this may occur because there are hundreds of millions of proliferating cirrhotic nodules, all being potentially pre-malignant, and eventually one or more of the nodules develop new HCCs.

The inflammatory background

More than 80% of patients with HCC also have separate liver disease(s) that often profoundly affects future management options. Most commonly this disease is associated with chronic inflammation (from HBV, HCV, or alcoholism, for example), which may lead to cirrhosis, depending on the duration and intensity of the inflammation. Such inflammation may also lead to complete liver failure, for which only liver transplantation is an effective treatment. Depending on the severity of the underlying liver damage (inflammation/fibrosis/cirrhosis), the ability to do resection or perform any ablation beyond that is needed for a minimal size tumor could be compromised by the risk of subsequent liver failure after the contemplated intervention. This can also be true for any potentially hepatotoxic medical therapy, such as systemic chemotherapy or TACE, also called chemoembolization. Since many chemotherapeutics also damage the bone marrow where granulocytes and platelets are produced, this combination can produce clinical toxicities. Furthermore, cirrhosis is often associated with

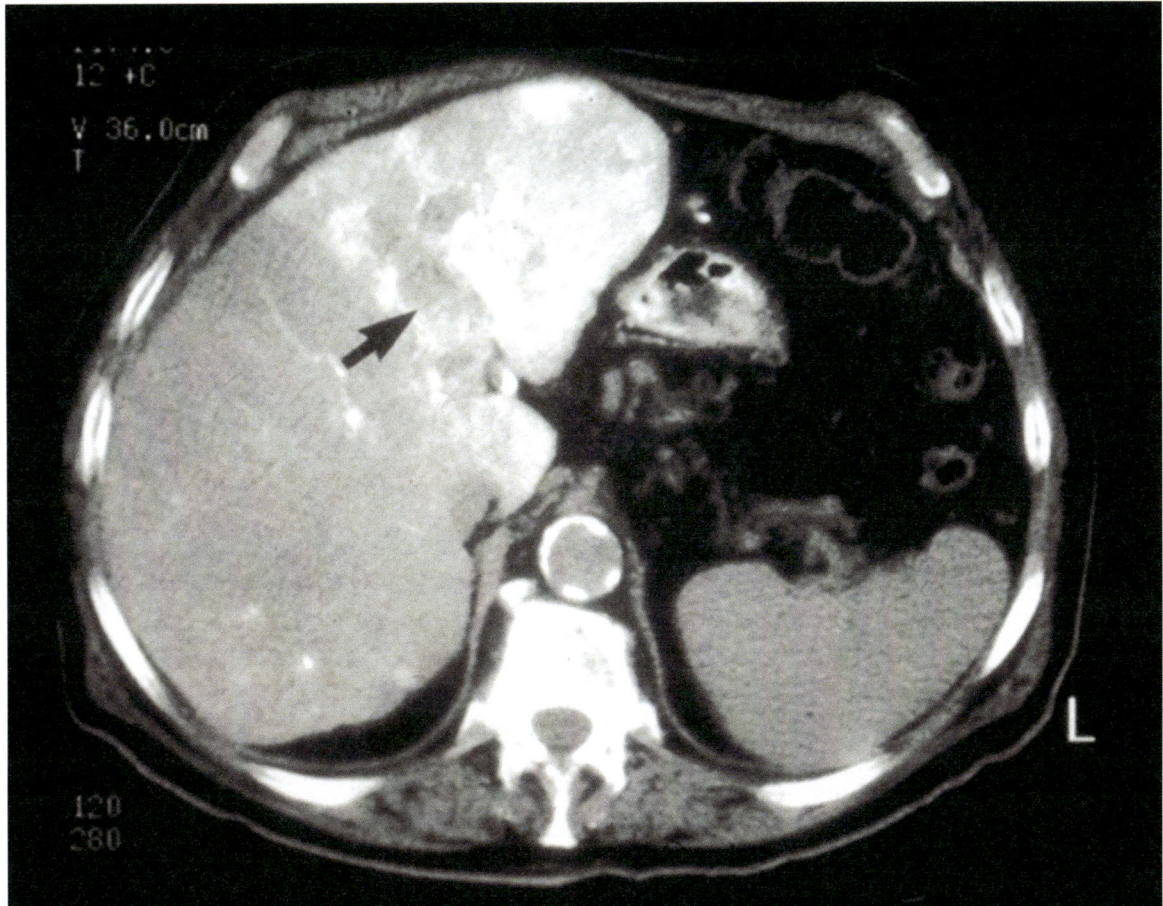

Figure 3 CAT scan showing vascularity and portal vein thrombosis (arrow) of hepatocellular carcinoma. Reproduced with permission from © Springer Science+Business Media, 2014; Carr BI. *Hepatocellular Carcinoma.* 2nd ed. New York, NY: Springer Science+Business Media; 2010.

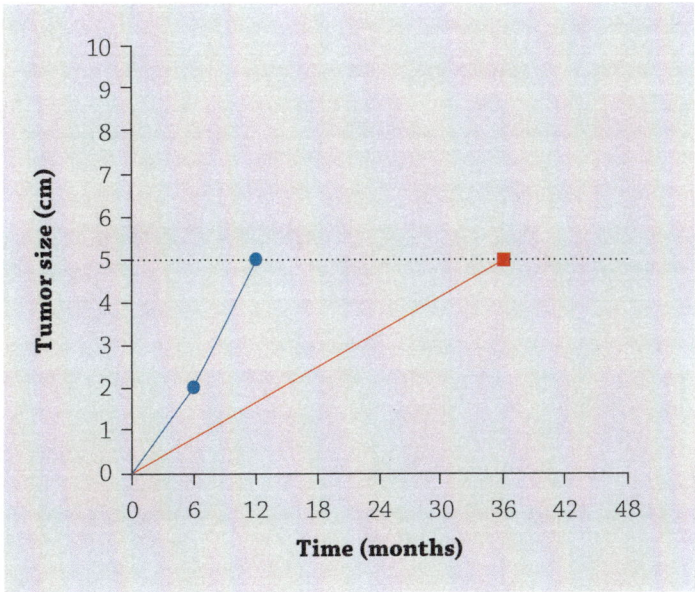

Figure 4 Varying growth rates of hepatocellular carcinoma.

bleeding tendencies from failure of the liver to produce sufficient coagulation proteins, in addition to low blood platelet counts thought to be due to splenic destruction of platelets from the back-pressure resulting from liver fibrosis. In summary, the fragility of the underlying liver can limit the safety of any therapy except liver transplantation.

Microenvironment

For several decades, it has been thought that tumors arise because one or more growth pathway genes become mutated and are expressed or otherwise activated in a way that leads to excessive stimulation of the growth control pathways of the cell; this is known as the oncogene hypothesis. There is much experimental support for this hypothesis; however, in recent years it has become clear that the activity of genes is often affected by other factors, either chemical controls on the gene involved, such as methylation, or by not yet well understood factors in their microenvironment (Table 5). Thus, both oxygenation and nutrients can affect how a given gene might behave within a cell, including oncogenes. Recent support for this "seed" (gene) and "soil" (cell environment) idea (a hypothesis originally developed for metastases by Stephen Paget) has come from molecular/clinical studies in which it has been found that the behavior of an HCC can be predicted from knowledge of the pattern of genetic changes (molecular signature) to be found in the nontumorous part of the liver. This environmental influence will have relevance in at least two HCC circumstances:

1. prediction of the behavior of an individual's tumor, such as the likelihood of recurrence after resection; and
2. the reason for the benefit of virus hepatitis therapy as part of HCC therapy in chronic virus carriers.

It has recently been shown that the high rates of recurrence after HCC resection can be significantly reduced, not by cancer therapeutics, but by antiviral therapy. Thus, the viral-mediated inflammation

1	**Pathophysiological processes: inflammation, fibrosis, angiogenesis**	
2	**Stromal cells: stellate cells (produce collagen and fibrosis), fibroblasts (involved in matrix), immune cells (lymphocytes and macrophages), angiogenic endothelial cells, platelets, gut bacteria/microbiota, stem cells/progenitor cells**	
3	**Stroma-derived growth and signaling molecules**	
a	Extracellular matrix proteins: fibronectin, collagen IV, tenascin C, matrix metalloproteinases (tissue remodeling, tumor cell invasion)	
b	Vascularization/angiogenesis factors: VEGF, PDGF, FGF, TGFα	
c	Immune and inflammatory mediators: interleukins, chemokines, reactive oxygen molecules, PDL-1	
d	Platelets: VEGF, PDGF, FGF, serotonin	
4	**Some drugs being tested that inhibit some of these targets**	
	Drug	**Target**
	Brivanib	VEGFR2, FGFR1
	Linifanib	VEGFR1, PDGFR
	Ramucirumab	VEGFR2
	Cixutumumab	IGF-R1
	CT-011	PD 1 and 2
	PI-88	Heparanase, sulfatase
	Sirolimus	mTOR
	AMG386	Angiopoietin 1 and 2
	Tivantinib	c-Met

Table 5 Hepatocellular carcinoma microenvironment. FGF, fibroblast growth factor; FGFR, fibroblast growth factor receptor; IGF-R, insulin-like growth factor receptor; mTOR, mammalian target of rapamycin; PD, programmed death; PDGF, platelet-derived growth factor; PDGFR, platelet-derived growth factor receptor; PDL-1, programmed death ligand-1; TGFα, transforming growth factor alpha; VEGF, vascular endothelial growth factor; VEGFR, vascular endothelial growth factor receptor.

must influence the HCC behavior. In summary, there are at least two types of molecular signatures (patterns of genetic changes) and clinical prognostic factors in HCC: those of the tumor and those of the underlying liver.

It has become increasingly clear in recent years that the behavior of a given HCC, and thus the treatment approaches for a patient with HCC, depend on more than just the clinically observed tumor characteristics. This was in a real sense anticipated in the 1985 staging system of the Japanese hepatologist Kunio Okuda, who brought attention to the need to consider both tumor and liver characteristics in prognosis and therapy. More recently, this approach has been greatly expanded by advances in HCC biology, biochemistry, and molecular understanding. As a result, a fuller understanding of HCC behavior needs to consider genes and gene alterations, tumor stroma (the underlying tissues), tumor neovasculature (the growth of new blood vessels that is necessary to support the increasing mass of the growing tumor), inflammation, supporting liver parenchyma (cells in the liver that support the specialized hepatocytes), and gene/molecular signatures (patterns of genes and their expression through proteins). Although much of this is still in the research realm (at least for the vasculature, inflammation, and molecular signatures), there is rapidly advancing clinical application. For example, new knowledge of the growth factors that encourage new blood vessel growth has led to the development of several new cancer drugs that target this vasculature, such as bevacizumab or sorafenib. Another example is the use of antihepatitis therapy to control HCC recurrences after successful resection.

Summary for patients, families, and caregivers

Understanding how HCC develops and progresses can help determine the best treatment options for the patient.

- Most people with HCC also have separate liver diseases, such as inflammation of the liver (hepatitis), scarred liver tissue (cirrhosis), or both. The severity of these diseases influences the patient's treatment choices. For example, a patient's diseased liver may be too fragile to safely treat the HCC with anticancer drugs. In this case, the patient's only option may be liver transplantation.

- Liver cancer cells can become resistant to the effects of anticancer drugs, such as chemotherapy. Giving these drugs, even at high doses, may have no effect for patients whose cells are resistant. The drugs can also be dangerous for their liver.

- The way blood travels in and out of the liver can also affect the development and treatment of a patient's HCC.
  - HCC tends to grow in the liver's blood vessels, and this may help cancerous cells enter the bloodstream and grow within other areas of the body.
  - Drugs and chemotherapy can sometimes be delivered directly into the cancer without affecting the rest of the liver.

- HCC cells grow at different rates: tumors that grow faster are associated with worse disease. Faster growing cancers can grow and spread around the surrounding liver, causing more lesions and tumors. It is important for patients to have repeated scans done to monitor how fast their tumors are growing.

- In recent years, there has been much progress in understanding HCC's structure, development, genetics, and how this relates to the patient's underlying liver disease. This has led to the development of new drugs and approaches for treating the disease.

Further reading

1   Hosaka T, Suzuki F, Kobayashi M, et al. Long-term entecavir treatment reduces hepatocellular carcinoma incidence in patients with hepatitis B virus infection. *Hepatology.* 2013;58:98-107.

2   Hsu YC, Ho HJ, Wu MS, Lin JT, Wu CY. Postoperative peg-interferon plus ribavirin is associated with reduced recurrence of hepatitis C virus-related hepatocellular carcinoma. *Hepatology.* 2013;58:150-157.

3 Wu SD, Ma YS, Fang Y, Liu LL, Fu D, Shen XZ. Role of the microenvironment in hepatocellular carcinoma development and progression. *Cancer Treat Rev.* 2012;38:218-225.

4 Yang JD, Nakamura I, Roberts LR. The tumor microenvironment in hepatocellular carcinoma: current status and therapeutic targets. *Semin Cancer Biol.* 2011;21:35-43.

5 Hernandez-Gea V, Toffanin S, Friedman SL, Llovet JM. Role of the microenvironment in the pathogenesis and treatment of hepatocellular carcinoma. *Gastroenterology.* 2013;144:512-527.

6 Carr BI, Guerra V. HCC and its microenvironment. *Hepatogastroenterology.* 2013;60:1433-1437.

7 Paget S. The distribution of secondary growths in cancer of the breast. 1889. *Cancer Metastasis Rev.* 1989;8:98-101.

8 Kinoshita A, Onoda H, Imai N, et al. The Glasgow Prognostic Score, an inflammation based prognostic score, predicts survival in patients with hepatocellular carcinoma. *BMC Cancer.* 2013;13:52.

9 Carr BI, Laishes BA. Carcinogen-induced drug resistance in rat hepatocytes. *Cancer Res.* 1981;41:1715-1719.

10 Haddow A. Cellular inhibition and the origin of cancer. *Acta Unio Int Concra Cancer.* 1938;3:342-352.

11 Carr BI, Guerra V, Giannini EG, et al; Italian Liver Cancer (ITA.LI.CA) Group. Association of abnormal plasma bilirubin with aggressive hepatocellular carcinoma phenotype. *Semin Oncol.* 2014;41:252-258.

Section 2

Clinical disease evaluation

Diagnosis A: Radiology

Ultrasound abdominal scanning is used widely for screening, as it is inexpensive and available in most countries. More definitive evaluation is then often needed for diagnosis, after a suspicious liver nodule is found on screening ultrasound, and is provided by a computed tomography (CT) or magnetic resonance imaging (MRI) scan. To a large extent the choice in the USA depends on the interest and expertise in a given institution. Recently introduced new MRI imaging agents have made this modality excellent for characterization of small lesions, especially those <1.5 cm diameter. These agents include super-paramagnetic iron oxide particles, which are taken up by Kupffer cells, and Gd-EOB-DTPA (gadolinium), which is taken up by hepatocytes, provides dynamic and liver-specific MRI images and is highly liver-specific. Hepatocellular carcinoma (HCC) diagnosis is frequently established by imaging criteria alone, based on the CT or MRI contrast enhancement pattern, with an intense contrast dye uptake by the suspected liver mass in the arterial phase followed by contrast washout in the venous, delayed phase. Many authorities in the field have recommended diagnosis on the scan alone if it has characteristic HCC appearances, without the need for biopsy, which is unlike the practice in all other cancers. This recommendation is based on the safety, sensitivity, and specificity of scans in HCCs ≥1.5 cm diameter, especially with "typical features" as well as the low, but present possibility of side effects from biopsy. Of course, atypical vascular lesions have always required biopsy. However, the increasing use of molecular markers (signatures) in oncology is likely to oblige a return to routine biopsy, as these molecular tools require tissue and are becoming mainstream clinical practice for many tumor types. Routinely on a first clinic evaluation, a chest CT is also performed to rule out the presence of lung metastases.

Summary for patients, families, and caregivers

Diagnosis for HCC begins by scanning a patient with imaging tests. For patients with possible HCC, an ultrasound scan of the abdomen is often used for screening. If the physician finds something suspicious on the ultrasound scan, a computed tomography (CT) or a magnetic resonance imaging (MRI) scan can be used to get a more definitive diagnosis. CT scans are also used to check if the cancer has spread to the lungs. A biopsy may be performed as well if the physician finds unusual lesions on the scans.

Further reading

1 Tan CH, Low S-C A, Thng CH. APASL and AASLD Consensus Guidelines on Imaging Diagnosis of Hepatocellular Carcinoma: A Review. *Int J Hepatol.* 2011;2011:519783.
2 Arii S, Sata M, Sakamoto M, et al. Management of hepatocellular carcinoma: Report of Consensus Meeting in the 45th Annual Meeting of the Japan Society of Hepatology (2009). *Hepatol Res.* 2010;40:667-685.
3 Di Martino M, De Filippis G, De Santis A, et al. Hepatocellular carcinoma in cirrhotic patients: prospective comparison of US, CT and MR imaging. *Eur Radiol.* 2013;23:887-896.

B. I. Carr, *Understanding Liver Cancer*, DOI: 10.1007/978-1-910315-02-6_2,
© Springer Healthcare 2014

Diagnosis B: Blood tests, tumor markers

While alpha-fetoprotein (AFP) is frequently used, inexpensive and is a simple blood test to use, it is elevated in only 50% of patients with HCC. AFP is not too sensitive a marker for screening for small, new HCCs (see page 10), but is extremely useful when following the response of an individual patient to therapy or to see if therapy fails. It is also beneficial when used after surgery, resection, or ablation for tracking the possibility of recurrence.

Recently, more HCC-specific tests have come into general clinical practice, such as a glycosylated form of AFP (itself, a fetal form of albumin) called AFP-L3 as well as des-gamma carboxy prothrombin (DCP). US Food and Drug Administration (FDA)-approved kits for measuring both AFP-L3 and DCP are readily available to physicians. Several studies have shown that elevated DCP is common in the presence of portal vein thrombosis (PVT). The molecule is really interesting, as it is an immature form of the coagulation protein, prothrombin. The enzyme responsible for catalyzing the immature to the mature form of prothrombin has an absolute requirement for vitamin K. This highlights an important role for vitamin K in HCC development.

Newer hepatocellular carcinoma tumor markers, proteomics, circulating tumor cells, and circulating DNA

Several new tumor markers are currently being evaluated, but do not yet have a place in routine clinical care. Tumor and liver molecular profiles or signatures were mentioned in the biology section of this book (see page 11). They have entered routine clinical practice for both prognosis and medical therapy selection for colorectal cancer, bronchogenic carcinoma, and melanoma, and are only at the validation stage for HCC. Unlike several other cancers for which single molecular markers are used, it seems that HCC may require a combination of markers or a molecular "signature".

The recent identification of HCC stem or progenitor cells and their characteristics, including epithelial cell adhesion molecule, cluster of differentiation 133, and cluster of differentiation 90 among others, offer the possibility of identifying specific HCC phenotypes and of targeting the stem cells for therapy. Keratin 19 has also been proposed as an invasive stem-cell marker.

Circulating tumor cells have recently been found in the blood of patients with different tumor types, including HCC, and are a valuable source for molecular genomics and proteomics analyses, without the need for a tumor biopsy to provide the material for this information. This is similarly true for circulating DNA. Newer markers that are currently being evaluated include miRNAs that are thought to be important in controlling cell behavior as well as newly studied serum proteins, including Glypican 3, angiopoietin 2, and vascular endothelial growth factor.

The importance of the microenvironment in HCC (see pages 14–15) has led to proposals that simple blood test estimates of inflammation are important patient prognosticators.

Summary for patients, families, and caregivers

Blood tests may be used to help detect HCC before or after surgery. Blood tests can also determine if therapy is working. Some blood tests for HCC include: alpha-fetoprotein (AFP) test, AFP-L3 test, and des-gamma carboxy prothrombin test.

Tumor markers are substances that can be found in the body that can indicate if a patient has cancer. For HCC, a combination of markers may be needed for a diagnosis. Researchers are still studying tumor markers to help healthcare teams diagnose HCC.

Further reading

1 Xu C, Yan Z, Zhou L, Wang Y. A comparison of glypican-3 with alpha-fetoprotein as a serum marker for hepatocellular carcinoma: a meta-analysis. *J Cancer Res Clin Oncol.* 2013;139:1417-1424.

2 Ertle JM, Heider D, Wichert M, et al. A combination of α-fetoprotein and des-γ-carboxy prothrombin is superior in detection of hepatocellular carcinoma. *Digestion.* 2013;87:121-131.

3 Bertino G, Ardiri AM, Calvagno GS, Bertino N, Boemi PM. Prognostic and diagnostic value of des-γ-carboxy prothrombin in liver cancer. *Drug News Perspect*. 2010;23:498-508.

4 Shirabe K, Itoh S, Yoshizumi T, et al. The predictors of microvascular invasion in candidates for liver transplantation with hepatocellular carcinoma—with special reference to the serum levels of des-gamma-carboxy prothrombin. *J Surg Oncol*. 2007;95:235-240.

5 Kim HS, Park JW, Jang JS, et al. Prognostic values of alpha-fetoprotein and protein induced by vitamin K absence or antagonist-II in hepatitis B virus-related hepatocellular carcinoma: a prospective study. *J Clin Gastroenterol*. 2009;43:482-488.

6 Mínguez B, Lachenmayer A. Diagnostic and prognostic molecular markers in hepatocellular carcinoma. *Dis Markers*. 2011;31:181-190.

7 Schröder PC, Segura V, Riezu JI, et al. A signature of six genes highlights defects on cell growth and specific metabolic pathways in murine and human hepatocellular carcinoma. *Funct Integr Genomics*. 2011;11:419-429.

8 Nault JC, De Reyniès A, Villanueva A, et al. A hepatocellular carcinoma 5-gene score associated with survival of patients after liver resection. *Gastroenterology*. 2013;145:176-187.

9 Borel F, Konstantinova P, Jansen PL. Diagnostic and therapeutic potential of miRNA signatures in patients with hepatocellular carcinoma. *J Hepatol*. 2012;56:1371-1383.

10 Nel I, Baba HA, Ertle J, et al. Individual profiling of circulating tumor cell composition and therapeutic outcome in patients with hepatocellular carcinoma. *Transl Oncol*. 2013;6:420-428.

11 Schulze K, Gasch C, Staufer K, et al. Presence of EpCAM-positive circulating tumor cells as biomarker for systemic disease strongly correlates to survival in patients with hepatocellular carcinoma. *Int J Cancer*. 2013;133:2165-2171.

12 Llovet JM, Peña CE, Lathia CD, Shan M, Meinhardt G, Bruix J; SHARP Investigators Study Group. Plasma biomarkers as predictors of outcome in patients with advanced hepatocellular carcinoma. *Clin Cancer Res*. 2012;18:2290-2300.

13 Pinato DJ, Stebbing J, Ishizuka M, et al. A novel and validated prognostic index in hepatocellular carcinoma: the inflammation based index (IBI). *J Hepatol*. 2012;57:1013-1020.

Diagnosis C: Biopsy – a debate

An HCC diagnosis is frequently made with considerable confidence based on the imaging characteristics alone of an arterial phase enhancing (vascular) mass with venous phase washout on CT or MRI scan. However, the standard of oncology care, especially for entry to clinical trials, usually requires the certainty of diagnosis that only a biopsy can provide. Furthermore, in this new age of proteomics for prognostication and treatment selection, a sample of tissue is usually required. Biopsy is a safe procedure in experienced hands, especially in the absence of ascites and where the tumor nodule is not in contact with an intrahepatic vessel. The benefits are certain diagnosis, especially when the radiological characteristics are not typical for HCC or the AFP levels are low. Risks include a slight risk of bleeding and the possibility of the tumor "seeding" into the biopsy needle track. This author's experience has shown a tumor seeding rate of 1%, and other reports show a tumor seeding rate of <5%. By not doing a biopsy, there is a risk of not having a correct diagnosis and then proceeding with potentially toxic or invasive therapy unnecessarily. Thus, with borderline cases based on clinical and radiological features, biopsy is needed. This whole argument may become moot if histological features or tissue becomes necessary for proteomics or genomics guidance for treatment choice, or if assay of circulating tumor cells becomes routine.

Further reading

1   Garrett R. Solid liver masses: approach to management from the standpoint of a radiologist. *Curr Gastroenterol Rep.* 2013;15:359.

2   Wee A. Fine-needle aspiration biopsy of hepatocellular carcinoma and related hepatocellular nodular lesions in cirrhosis: controversies, challenges, and expectations. *Patholog Res Int.* 2011;2011:587936.

Assessment of tumor extent for treatment planning: staging classifications

Functional hepatic reserve, Child-Pugh classification

As previously discussed, patients are grouped by definition into three categories of liver damage severity (A, B, or C), according to the Child-Pugh (CP) classification cirrhosis score (see Table 3). A patient classified as CP A has essentially normal liver function and can receive almost any therapy without extra risk resulting from their liver disease. They typically have a 100% 12-month survival, without HCC or any treatment. Patients who are classified as CP C have poor liver function and can only receive liver transplant. Without transplant, their survival is typically 40% at 12 months, with or without HCC. Patients with a CP B score are a heterogeneous group. At one end, they approach CP C and need great caution in being given therapies. At the other end, they can have quite good liver function and can tolerate many medical therapies, some ablative therapies, and minor resection. They typically have a 60% 12-month survival, without HCC and without treatment. As shown in Figure 4 (page 13), patients can have varied liver disease severity and tumor characteristics across the classification spectrum.

Integrated tumor and liver function staging

Several classification systems have been proposed that integrate both liver prognostic features and HCC characteristics. At this time, two systems are widely used in Europe and the USA, and one in Japan. In Europe, both the Cancer of the Liver Italian Program (CLIP) score and the Barcelona Clinic Liver Cancer (BCLC) system are commonly used; in Japan, the Japan Integrated Staging (JIS) score has received consensus recognition. Other scoring systems have been proposed from Japan, France, Hong Kong, and elsewhere, but they all share the features of integrating both adverse liver and adverse tumor characteristics. Thus, they all incorporate CP liver function features, as well as tumor size and number and presence of PVT. Their purpose is two-fold, namely prognosis and treatment selection. In summary, adverse prognostic factors are:

A.   Tumor factors: large size, multiple tumor nodules, diffuse tumor, presence of PVT, high blood AFP levels, presence of metastases.

B.   Liver factors: high blood bilirubin, aspartate aminotransferase/alanine transaminase, gamma-glutamyl transpeptidase levels; low blood albumin and low platelet levels (the latter a reflection of severity of cirrhosis) and presence of more than minimal ascites.

C.   However, in addition, good prognosis macroenvironmental factors include being female, age >75 years, and especially the combination of both.

D.   Recently, indices of inflammation have been recognized and accepted as important prognostic markers. The most prominent of these is the C-reactive protein and albumin protein blood test (Glasgow Prognostic Score).

Summary for patients, families, and caregivers

To choose the right treatment for a patient, the healthcare team must know the severity of the patient's liver disease. Healthcare teams use the Child-Pugh score to determine the severity of the patient's liver disease. This score consists of three categories of liver damage: A, B, and C:

- Patients with a **Child-Pugh A** score have almost normal liver function. They can receive almost any type of treatment.
- Patients with a **Child-Pugh B** score are treated depending how close they are to a Child-Pugh A or C score.
- Patients with a **Child-Pugh C** score have very poor liver function. They almost always require a liver transplant.

Additionally, comprehensive classification systems combine an assessment of the Child-Pugh score, liver factors, gender, age, tumor size and how far the tumor has spread throughout the body. The combined assessments can help determine possible treatment approaches and how a patient's disease might develop.

Further reading

1 Kinoshita A, Onoda H, Imai N, et al. The Glasgow Prognostic Score, an inflammation based prognostic score, predicts survival in patients with hepatocellular carcinoma. *BMC Cancer.* 2013;13:52.

2 Cabibbo G, Maida M, Genco C, et al. Natural history of untreatable hepatocellular carcinoma: A retrospective cohort study. *World J Hepatol.* 2012;4:256-261.

3 Sirivatanauksorn Y, Tovikkai C. Comparison of staging systems of hepatocellular carcinoma. *HPB Surg.* 2011;2011:818217

4 Hsu CY, Hsia CY, Huang YH, et al. Selecting an optimal staging system for hepatocellular carcinoma: comparison of 5 currently used prognostic models. *Cancer.* 2010;116:3006-3014.

5 Huitzil-Melendez FD, Capanu M, O'Reilly EM, et al. Advanced hepatocellular carcinoma: which staging systems best predict prognosis? *J Clin Oncol.* 2010;28:2889-2895.

6 Marrero JA, Kudo M, Bronowicki JP. The challenge of prognosis and staging for hepatocellular carcinoma. *Oncologist.* 2010;15 Suppl 4:23-33.

7 Carr BI, Buch SC, Kondragunta V, Pancoska P, Branch RA. Tumor and liver determinants of prognosis in unresectable hepatocellular carcinoma: a case cohort study. *J Gastroenterol Hepatol.* 2008;23:1259-1266.

8 Shiba H, Furukawa K, Fujiwara Y, et al. Postoperative peak serum C-reactive protein predicts outcome of hepatic resection for hepatocellular carcinoma. *Anticancer Res.* 2013;33:705-709.

9 Zhang JF, Shu ZJ, Xie CY, et al. Prognosis of unresectable hepatocellular carcinoma: comparison of seven staging systems (TNM, Okuda, BCLC, CLIP, CUPI, JIS, CIS) in a Chinese cohort. *PLoS One.* 2014;9:e88182.

The new patient assessment

The following section will review the clinical evaluation and examination of a new patient with possible HCC. Tables 6 and 7 summarize the clinical presentation, symptoms, and evaluation discussed further in this section.

Medical history and physical examination

The history is important in evaluating putative predisposing factors, including a history of hepatitis or jaundice, blood transfusion, or use of intravenous drugs. A family history of HCC or hepatitis should be sought and a detailed social history taken to include job descriptions for industrial exposure to possible carcinogenic compounds. Physical examination should include assessing stigmata of underlying liver disease, such as jaundice (seen as yellowness in the sclera or white part of the eyes), ascites (abdominal fluid), peripheral edema (leg swelling), spider nevi, palmar erythema (hand redness), and weight loss. Evaluation of the abdomen for hepatic size, masses or ascites, hepatic nodularity and tenderness, and splenomegaly is needed, as is assessment of overall performance status and psychosocial evaluation (Table 6). Basic physical exam includes pulse and blood pressure, and an assessment of whether the patient is clinically sick. Family support evaluation is important at this stage, especially if liver transplantation is being considered.

Blood tests

Blood tests typically include (Table 7):

1. Complete blood count, including hemoglobin, white cell count and platelet count, and prothrombin time (a test for blood coagulation ability).
2. Liver function tests: total bilirubin, albumin, gamma-glutamyl transpeptidase, alkaline phosphatase (ALKP), and the transaminases aspartate aminotransferase and alanine transaminase (serum glutamic oxaloacetic transaminase and serum glutamic-pyruvic transaminase), and cholesterol and serum iron levels.
3. Renal function tests: urea and creatinine.
4. HCC tumor markers: AFP, AFP-L3, and DCP.
5. Measurement of hepatitis C and B serology. If either is positive, more detailed virological measurements and body immune response measurements will need to be obtained.

Radiology

CT or MRI scan should be performed to obtain baseline, pre-therapy assessment of tumor maximum dimensions, tumor number, and location within the liver as well as proximity to main vessels, which will influence ablation approach. The radiology also permits identification of the presence of portal vein invasion or PVT, a major negative prognostic factor, and may allow discernment of the presence of cirrhosis if cirrhotic nodularity can be seen as well as of ascites.

Summary for patients, families, and caregivers
A person's medical history can provide important clues as to whether they are at risk for HCC. During a new patient assessment, the healthcare team may ask about the patient's social life and family history of cancer and liver diseases. They may also ask about the patient's work environment to see if they have been in contact with harmful chemicals at work. The healthcare team will perform a physical exam to record their basic health, check for swelling of the abdomen, look for yellow skin or eyes, and other characteristics that are signs of possible liver disease. They will also ask for blood tests and imaging tests. If a liver transplant might be needed in the future, the healthcare team may also see if the patient has support from their families.

Symptom	% of patients
No symptom	30
Abdominal pain	40
Routine physical examination finding, abnormal liver blood tests	24
Weight loss	20
Cirrhosis symptoms (ankle swelling, abdominal bloating, increased girth-fluid or liver, pruritus, gastrointestinal bleed)	20
Appetite loss	11
Other (evaluation of anemia and various diseases)	12
Routine CT scan screening of known cirrhosis	17
Weakness/malaise	15
Jaundice and itching	5
Jaundice	5
Tumor rupture (mainly in Africa)	1

Table 6 Clinical presentation and symptoms. CT, computed tomography scan. Adapted from © McGraw-Hill Global Education Holdings, LLC, 2014; Carr BI. Chapter 92. Tumors of the Liver and Biliary Tree. In: Longo DL, Fauci AS, Kasper DL, et al, eds. *Harrison's Principles of Internal Medicine.* 18th edition. New York, NY: The McGraw-Hill Companies, Inc; 2012.

1	Blood tests: full blood count (splenomegaly), liver function tests, ammonia levels, electrolytes, AFP and DCP (PIVKA-2), Ca^{2+} and Mg^{2+}; hepatitis B, C, and D serology (and quantitative HBV DNA or HCV RNA if either is positive); neurotensin (specific for fibrolamellar HCC)
2	Triphasic dynamic helical (spiral) CT scan of liver (or MRI scan); chest CT scan; upper and lower gastrointestinal endoscopy (for varices, bleeding, ulcers); and brain scan (only if symptoms suggest)
3	Core biopsy: of the tumor and separate biopsy of the underlying liver

Table 7 Clinical evaluation. AFP, alpha fetoprotein; CT, computed tomography scan; DCP, des-gamma carboxy prothrombin; HBV, hepatitis B virus; HCC, hepatocellular carcinoma; HCV, hepatitis C virus; MRI, magnetic resonance imaging scan. Adapted from © McGraw-Hill Global Education Holdings, LLC, 2014; Carr BI. Chapter 92. Tumors of the Liver and Biliary Tree. In: Longo DL, Fauci AS, Kasper DL, et al, eds. *Harrison's Principles of Internal Medicine.* 18th edition. New York, NY: The McGraw-Hill Companies, Inc; 2012.

Further Reading

1 Carr BI. Chapter 92. Tumors of the Liver and Biliary Tree. In: Longo DL, Fauci AS, Kasper DL, et al, eds. *Harrison's Principles of Internal Medicine.* 18th edition. New York, NY: The McGraw-Hill Companies, Inc; 2012:777-785.

2 Carr BI. Chapter 111. Tumors of the Liver and Biliary Tree. In: Longo DL, Fauci AS, Kasper DL, et al, eds. *Harrison's Principles of Internal Medicine.* 19th edition. New York, NY: The McGraw-Hill Companies, Inc; 2014: in press.

Section 3

Management of hepatocellular carcinoma

Both the prognosis and the selection of the type of therapy depend upon three factors, which themselves may be interacting:

1. the extent of the tumor (hepatocellular carcinoma [HCC]),
2. the aggressiveness (biology) of the tumor, and
3. the degree of liver dysfunction (hepatitis or cirrhosis or both).

Furthermore, the therapy may also impact both the liver dysfunction (hepatotoxic effects of chemotherapy) as well as any residual microscopic tumor (immunosuppression after liver transplantation or effects of liver regeneration after resection on micrometastases). A list of treatment options for HCC is summarized in Table 8.

Surgery
Resection
Liver transplantation
Local ablative therapies
Cryosurgery
Radiofrequency ablation
Microwave ablation
Percutaneous ethanol injection
Regional therapies: Hepatic artery transcatheter treatments
Transarterial chemotherapy
Transarterial embolization
Transarterial chemoembolization
Transarterial drug-eluting beads
Transarterial radiotherapies (internal liver radiation)
^{90}Yttrium microspheres
^{131}Iodine-ethiodol
External beam radiation for portal vein thrombosis
Conformal external beam radiation
Systemic therapies
Molecularly targeted therapies (eg, sorafenib)
Chemotherapy
Immunotherapy
Hormonal therapy
Supportive therapies

Table 8 Summary of treatment options for hepatocellular carcinoma. Reproduced with permission from © Springer Science+Business Media, 2014; Carr BI. *Hepatocellular Carcinoma.* 2nd ed. New York, NY: Springer Science+Business Media; 2010.

B. I. Carr, *Understanding Liver Cancer*, DOI: 10.1007/978-1-910315-02-6_3,
© Springer Healthcare 2014

25

The therapies associated with the longest survival (in years) include the three "surgical" approaches of (1) tumor ablation or killing (radiofrequency ablation [RFA] or other ablative therapies, such as microwave ablation [MWA], percutaneous ethanol injection, cryotherapy, or hyperthermia), (2) surgical resection, or (3) liver transplantation.

The intent of the ablative therapies, such as RFA, which are minimally invasive (unlike resection surgery), is to kill or "sterilize" the cells in the tumor mass by use of a probe to kill them with radiofrequency or microwaves, by cold, heat, or chemical means (alcohol in percutaneous ethanol injection). Ablation is most effective for tumors ≤3 cm maximum diameter. Various probes and techniques claim effectiveness up to or equal to 5 cm diameter. Beyond 5 cm, the effectiveness appears to diminish, and classical resection surgery is used. Resection can also be used for any size of technically resectable HCC. However, both ablative therapies and resection also face certain limitations. The main one is the severity of the underlying cirrhosis. This is because a rim of normal liver needs to be included with the resected tumor (the surgeon's eyes can only see visible but not microscopic tumor), the amount of liver that is surgically removed has the potential to cause irreversible liver failure in the remnant liver in patients with cirrhosis, as the remaining liver may not be able to support the metabolic needs and life of the patient. Ablation, which uses liver probes to deliver radiofrequency waves, microwaves, heat or cold, often does not have this problem. However, another risk with ablation is the topology of the tumor within the liver. If the HCC is adjacent to a major liver blood vessel or bile duct, then major liver damage can occur with attempts to ablate or resect the tumor mass. Both of these issues are avoided by treatment with liver transplantation, as this is the only therapy that can cure two diseases at once; namely, both the HCC and the underlying liver disease. For patients whose tumor(s) cannot be resected or ablated or who do not fit within the transplant criteria of one lesion ≤5 cm or 3 lesions none >3 cm (see liver transplant section [page 32]), then the treatment choices are medical; however, some of these treatments, such as transarterial chemoembolization (TACE) also called "chemoembolization", can cause a decrease in tumor size, permitting reconsideration of RFA, resection, or liver transplantation after a therapy-induced size decrease. No systemic (oral or intravenous) chemotherapy has thus far been shown to confer any survival advantage compared with no treatment, although chemoembolization can increase survival.

It was discovered several decades ago that whereas most internal organs receive their oxygenated blood by a feeding artery and have the deoxygenated blood removed by a vein, the situation in the liver is more complex. The normal liver receives about 75% of its total blood flow from the portal vein, but only about 55% of its oxygen supply from this source, as the intestines remove oxygen from it first. The remaining 45% of oxygenated blood comes from the hepatic artery. By contrast, HCCs receive their oxygenated blood predominantly from hepatic artery branches, with exceptions being very well differentiated HCCs. As a result, it was found that HCC therapies could be delivered to the tumor(s) via injection or infusion into the hepatic artery or a branch artery in a clinic setting, with relative sparing of the underlying liver. This permits relatively selective treatment of the HCC with high doses of directed therapy, with considerable sparing of the underlying liver from treatment toxicities and even more sparing of the rest of the body, as the therapy is taken up by the tumor and to a lesser extent by the liver. This is the main rationale behind hepatic artery chemoembolization (TACE) and radioembolization (see page 34). These are the two main treatments for non-metastatic HCC that cannot be ablated, resected, or transplanted. Several forms of systemic hormonal therapy have been tried and shown to be minimally effective.

The oral therapy sorafenib (marketed as NEXAVAR®, Bayer HealthCare Pharmaceuticals Inc., Whippany, NJ, USA; Onyx Pharmaceuticals, Inc., San Francisco, CA, USA; a multikinase inhibitor that antagonizes tumor cell proliferation and angiogenesis) has been given US Food and Drug Administration (FDA) approval for treating HCC. It modestly enhances survival, despite minimal tumor shrinkage and considerable toxicity, which will be further discussed on page 37. Its main use is after failure of TACE/chemoembolization, after failure of radioembolization, if TACE/chemoembolization or radioembolization are unsafe, or for metastatic HCC. Because TACE/chemoembolization shrinks tumors and can enhance survival, and sorafenib enhances survival by quite different means, there are now a number of ongoing studies to evaluate the combination of sorafenib with other therapies, including TACE/chemoembolization, resection, RFA, transplant, and radioembolization (see pages 27–44). Furthermore, TACE/chemoembolization, radioembolization, and sorafenib are treatment options as "bridge to transplant" for patients awaiting liver transplantation whose tumors need to be kept stable for them to stay on the transplant waiting list (if their tumors grow, they often cannot be considered transplant recipients).

In addition, clinical trials are evaluating the efficacy of many other kinase inhibitors and growth inhibiting drugs with a variety of mechanisms of action; however, not all patients are eligible for receiving anti-HCC therapy. Some patients, especially those with a Child-Pugh (CP) classification cirrhosis score of C with overt liver failure, or with acute jaundice from acute portal vein thrombosis (PVT), cannot receive any of the above therapy approaches and need symptomatic or palliative care only.

A treatment algorithm for patients who have been diagnosed with HCC is described in Figure 5. Even within this treatment algorithm, each patient needs to be evaluated as an individual. Numerous factors and details must be taken into account by the treating physicians; these factors include the details of tumor size, number, and location within the liver, presence of regional lymph nodes or distant metastases, the degree of liver damage, plus the individual patient's affect, hopes, psychological make-up, and family support. For this reason, the idea of a multidisciplinary management team has proven to be popular and highly effective in recent years to assess the strengths and limitations of each treatment type for the needs of each individual patient, patient's tumor and liver setting. Additionally, the multidisciplinary team can evaluate the often cascade of treatments that need to be considered, which are commonly contingent on results of the previous therapeutic step.

Summary for patients, families, and caregivers
Treatment plans for patients with HCC are based on:
• How far the cancer has spread throughout the liver: size and number of cancer nodules
• How fast the cancer is growing and whether a scan has shown that cancer has grown in a critical vein of the liver, known as the portal vein
• How the liver is functioning
Patients should be evaluated and treated as unique individuals. The treatment should be tailored to their own specific needs and circumstances. A multidisciplinary team of various specialists should work together to help support the patient by evaluating each therapeutic step and reviewing the patient's tumor(s), liver disease, hopes, psychological make-up, and family support.

General treatment choices

There are three general groups of patients from the treatment choice perspective:

- **Group 1** - **Potentially curable. Treatment choices: ablation, resection, or transplantation**
- **Group 2** - **Treatable, with intent to prolong survival. Treatment choices: TACE/chemoembolization, radioembolization, kinase inhibitors (sorafenib)**
- **Group 3** - **Palliation. Treatment choice: symptom relief through palliative care for advanced disease**

The greatest effort is applied to identify patients suitable for Group 1 therapies, as described above.

The following section outlines a general list of treatment options, partially based on a mix of consensus recommendations from Japan, Europe, and the USA (ie, Japan Integrated Staging [JIS], European Organisation for Research and Treatment of Cancer [EORTC], and American Association for the Study of Liver Diseases [AASLD]) and from clinical practice, which varies widely, especially in regard to choice of ablative therapy.

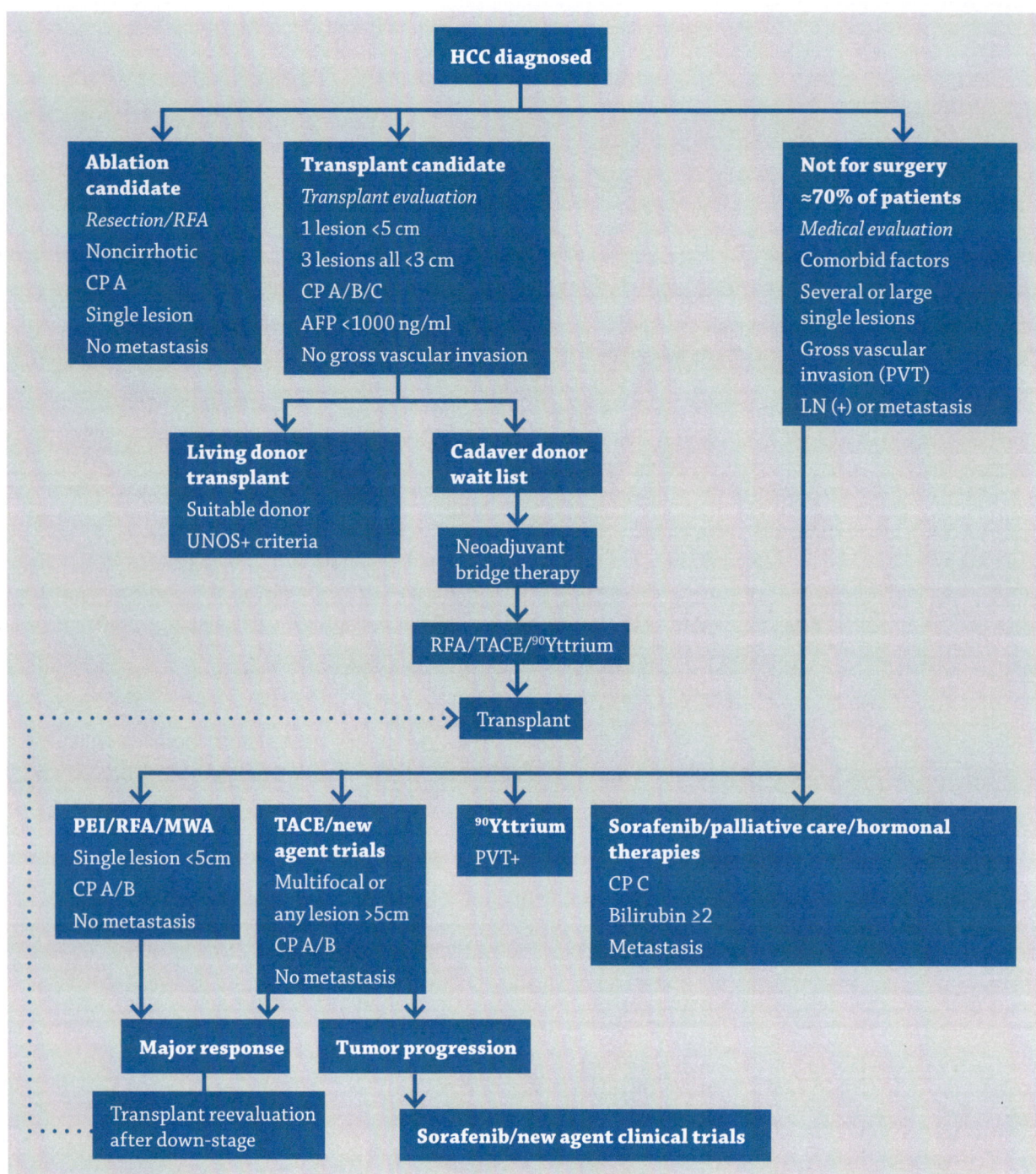

Figure 5 Treatment algorithm for patients with hepatocellular carcinoma. AFP, alpha-fetoprotein; CP, Child-Pugh cirrhosis score; HCC, hepatocellular carcinoma; LN, lymph node; MWA, microwave ablation; PEI, percutaneous ethanol injection; PVT, portal vein thrombosis; RFA, radiofrequency ablation; TACE, transarterial chemoembolization; UNOS, United Network for Organ Sharing.

There are five broad treatment approaches, each with its own general indications. The group numbers indicated below correspond with the three general groups of patients listed above.

- **Group 1. Ablation or resection*:** first choice for a small tumor with excellent liver function. Expected survival: 40–70% at 5 years, typically 50–60 months.

- **Group 1. Liver transplantation*:** first choice for a small number of tumors or a single tumor up to 6.5 cm diameter; can apply to any level of liver function. Expected survival: 70–80% at 5 years, typically 100+ months.

- **Group 2. Hepatic arterial therapies (TACE/chemoembolization and radioembolization):** for large, widespread, or multiple tumors without metastases or PVT (but patients with PVT can receive radioembolization). Expected survival: 5–30% at 2 years, typically 24–36 months.

- **Group 2. Systemic therapy, predominantly sorafenib:** for managing metastases, presence of PVT, or failed TACE/chemoembolization or radioembolization. Safe in patients with a CP cirrhosis score of A and for some patients with a CP B score. About 11 month median survival.

- **Group 3. Palliative, symptomatic care:** when none of the above can be offered or have failed. Expected survival: <3 months

*Only ablation, resection and transplantation are potentially curative (Group 1).

All decision making for treatment depends on the totality of a limited number of tumor and liver parameters, with two of them excluding curative therapies. These two are: presence of extra-hepatic metastases and presence of macroscopic (observable on CT or MRI scan) main PVT. Metastasis is a definitive exclusion criterion, whereas PVT may be relative, depending on its extent and how good the liver function is. Decision making is thus based on a series of exclusions (see list below). The list below follows general clinical practice guidelines only. There will likely be various combinations of tumor and liver abnormalities that only a multidisciplinary team can assess in its totality for any individual patient. For example, a single branch PVT in a ≤3 cm HCC, which is common, could be approached with resection, ablation, TACE/chemoembolization or radioembolization, or by resection alone for a >3 cm tumor mass.

1. The presence of distant metastasis usually excludes any surgery or regional therapy.
   - For patients with CP C cirrhosis score or the more severe forms of CP B, the treatment choice is palliative care.
   - For patients with good liver function CP A or mild dysfunction CP B, the choice is sorafenib or new systemic agents in cancer clinical trials (for further information, see www.clinicaltrials.gov).
   - Patients with CP C with or without metastases usually need palliative care. However, some patients with non-metastatic CP C can be considered for liver transplantation.

2. If the main portal vein is thrombosed/occluded (PVT), any ablation, resection, or liver transplantation is excluded. The treatment choices for these patients are sorafenib, radioembolization or palliative care (depending on their general condition and liver function).

3. For patients with right or left branch PVT, radioembolization has been shown to be relatively safe, but TACE/chemoembolization is less so. However, intrahepatic arterial chemotherapy without embolization is an option.

4. For patients with advanced tumors with large or multifocal tumor nodules exceeding the Milan criteria, the treatment choice depends on the severity of cirrhosis. The Milan criteria evaluates a patient's tumor(s) to determine whether the patient with HCC can benefit from a liver transplant. The Milan criteria state that a patient can be selected for and benefit from liver transplantation if the tumor number is ≤3, all with size ≤3 cm, or if the patient has a single tumor or lesion ≤5 cm (or possibly <6.5 cm), and will be discussed in more depth on page 32. For patients with CP A or B cirrhosis, the choices are TACE/chemoembolization,

radioembolization, or possibly a new drug in clinical trial. If the tumor grows while on these treatments, then the patient may be treated with sorafenib or a new agent. Some patients who have major tumor shrinkage on therapy may then be re-considered for liver transplantation.

5. Patients within Milan criteria, with any CP grade, can be considered for liver transplantation, psychosocial evaluation permitting. Thus, the use of liver transplantation is independent of any severity of cirrhosis. In addition, many patients within Milan criteria can also be treated by resection, RFA, or a combination of these, for CP A or for mild degrees of CP B cirrhosis.

6. A single large HCC of any size >5 cm without cirrhosis or with CP A may be considered for resection.

7. For small lesions ≤3 cm, the choices include resection or RFA, unless there are ≥4 lesions, in which case the patient is better treated with TACE/chemoembolization or radioembolization. Patients who respond to therapy with decrease in size or number of their tumors can always then be reconsidered for potentially curative RFA, resection, or liver transplantation. Similarly, patients whose tumors progress or recur after ablation/resection/TACE/chemoembolization or radioembolization can be considered for sorafenib or possibly a new agent as part of a clinical trial.

8. Whenever a new agent in clinical trial is suggested, it is usually because there is no standard of therapy known to enhance survival in that circumstance or to compare a new therapy to whatever is considered as "standard" therapy.

9. Some patients have small lesions with either a negative biopsy or non-hypervascularity on radiology scan. They are, therefore, atypical for HCC, and usually repetitive radiology/AFP follow up is recommended, often at 3-month intervals.

Summary for patients, families, and caregivers

When choosing a treatment for a patient, there are three general groups that patients fall into:

- **Group 1 – Patients who might be potentially cured.** Their liver tumor(s) is/are small in size and number and they have good liver function. These patients' treatment options include: killing/sterilizing the cancer cells (ablation), surgically removing the HCC (resection), or liver transplant. These are the only treatment options available that might cure the HCC.

- **Group 2 – Patients who are treatable, but with more advanced disease.** These patients may have tumors that are large, widespread within the liver, and/or multiple tumors in their liver. These patients' treatment options include receiving anticancer drugs (TACE/ chemoembolization or radioembolization). If these options do not work, then the multidisciplinary team can treat the patient with an oral medication called sorafenib, even in the presence of distant metastases.

- **Group 3 – Patients who have very advanced and widespread HCC or the previous treatments have failed.** These patients can be offered palliative care. Palliative care means that the healthcare team will focus on managing the patient's symptoms and providing the patient relief from pain and stress.

The multidisciplinary team should additionally work together to rule out treatment options based on unique circumstances that their patient may be experiencing. The team should educate the patient and their family/caregivers on various treatment options so they will be properly cared for and supported.

Further reading

1 Asayama Y, Yoshimitsu K, Nishihara Y, et al. Arterial blood supply of hepatocellular carcinoma and histologic grading: radiologic-pathologic correlation. *AJR Am J Roentgenol.* 2008;190:W28-W34.

2 Park JW, Amarapurkar D, Chao Y, et al. Consensus recommendations and review by an International Expert Panel on Interventionsin Hepatocellular Carcinoma (EPOIHCC). *Liver Int.* 2013;33:327-337.

3 Arii S, Sata M, Sakamoto M, et al. Management of hepatocellular carcinoma: Report of Consensus Meeting in the 45th Annual Meeting of the Japan Society of Hepatology (2009). *Hepatol Res.* 2010;40:667-685.

4 Poon D, Anderson BO, Chen LT, et al; Asian Oncology Summit. Management of hepatocellular carcinoma in Asia: consensus statement from the Asian Oncology Summit 2009. *Lancet Oncol.* 2009;10:1111-1118.

5 Kudo M, Izumi N, Kokudo N, et al; HCC Expert Panel of Japan Society of Hepatology. Management of hepatocellular carcinoma in Japan: Consensus-Based Clinical Practice Guidelines proposed by the Japan Society of Hepatology (JSH) 2010 updated version. *Dig Dis.* 2011;29:339-364.

6 European Association for Study of Liver; European Organisation for Research and Treatment of Cancer. EASL-EORTC clinical practice guidelines: management of hepatocellular carcinoma. *Eur J Cancer.* 2012;48:599-641.

Therapies with curative intent (Group 1)

Ablation (Group 1)
Ablation is the destruction or killing of cells in a tumor nodule, without its physical removal by surgery. Radiofrequency ablation (RFA) has come to be considered a standard of care for small lesions (normally ≤3 cm), since a small number of small lesions (usually 1–3) can be completely necrosed (killed) by the RFA instrument probe. Some newer probes have been promoted for larger single lesions up to 5 cm. Some other techniques, such as MWA and cryoablation (freezing), are being investigated. Around 10% of patients cannot be treated by RFA due to the location of the tumor(s) and these are often treated with ultrasound-guided alcohol injection (percutaneous ethanol injection). Recent reports show that for >5 cm lesions, the combination of RFA plus TACE/chemoembolization produces superior results in terms of decreases in recurrence.

Resection (Group 1)
The time-hallowed treatment has been **surgical resection**, either by open surgical technique or more recently by minimally invasive procedure. This is still the standard for single lesions ≥5 cm with normal liver function, CP A cirrhosis, or many cases with good function CP B cirrhosis. A variation has been to use therapeutic portal vein embolization on the tumor-bearing side of the liver, which often results in the expansion of the other, non-tumorous liver lobe, resulting in an increased amount of residual liver tissue after the procedure. Like TACE/chemoembolization, this is done by placing a needle through the skin and into the liver and into the blood vessel. It is done as a day procedure in the vascular radiology department. Resection of the lobe containing the HCC can then be done more safely, as the expanded remaining lobe has more liver mass to support the patient's metabolic needs. There are many reports of the use of resection in the absence of main trunk PVT, with variable survival being reported; some centers have reported operative mortality is <5% and 5-year survival is >50%, but with HCC recurrence ranging from 40–80%. Two types of HCC recurrence are recognized: early recurrence <12 months, likely from growth of microscopic residual HCC; and late recurrence, putatively from new HCCs being formed in the pre-malignant residual cirrhotic liver nodules. Many studies have been done of neo-adjuvant (before resection) and adjuvant (after resection) chemotherapies to try and reduce the incidence of HCC recurrence. So far, this approach has not been convincingly beneficial, although TACE/chemoembolization has been used to decrease tumor size or number to permit a subsequent resection to be performed. There are also many reports of second resections for tumor recurrence. Trials are currently ongoing to assess the usefulness of adjuvant sorafenib. A recent randomized trial of sorafenib in the post-resection adjuvant setting (STORM trial) unfortunately showed no added benefit for the addition of the drug to resected patients. TACE/chemoembolization added to RFA has been reported to have better outcomes when

combined than when RFA was used alone. Although chemotherapy has not been shown to decrease recurrence rates post-resection, antiviral HCV therapy with peg-interferon plus ribavirin has recently been shown to decrease recurrences. This seems to be a therapeutic major advance. Some patients with potentially resectable HCC cannot be resected, however, due to the severity of their underlying liver damage. The reason is that each person's liver is appropriate to their metabolic needs. The normal liver is an organ that can regenerate or replenish itself, if part is removed or damaged. The surgeon depends on this regeneration of the liver for patient survival post-resection. However, the liver that is chronically damaged, as is typical of chronic hepatitis or cirrhosis, often cannot regenerate itself sufficiently for safe surgery.

Liver transplantation (Group 1)

Liver transplantation for HCC has been evaluated for 30 years. It is the only therapy with the potential to cure both the HCC and the cirrhosis at the same time. There were two aims for liver transplantation and HCC: (1) to permit the surgeon to remove the tumor no matter how severe the cirrhosis, which often proves to be successful in clinical practice; and (2) to extend the ability of the surgeon to remove ever larger tumors; this second aim has proven to be of limited benefit due to the high recurrence rate when large HCCs or those associated with PVT are treated with liver transplantation. Considering that livers for liver transplantation are a limited resource, the idea has gained general acceptance that they should be used for patients with HCC only when the expected survival is similar to that with patients without cancer. The Milan criteria have been used since 1996, with a 5-year survival rate of around 75% for single HCCs ≤5 cm or up to 3 lesions, each lesion ≤3 cm. However, this standard has been found to be restrictive, and other recommendations, such as the University of California San Francisco (UCSF) criteria, have recently found support for similar post-transplant survival rates with a single lesion ≤6.5 cm or ≤3 nodules with the largest lesion to be no more than 4.5 cm and combined tumor diameter of all lesions <8 cm. Given that hepatitis often recurs in the new, transplanted liver, aggressive post-operative antiviral regimens are used. More recently, it has been found that patients aged >65 years or within the Milan criteria tumors in patients with blood AFP levels >1000 ng/ml do particularly badly and such patients are restricted from liver transplantation, unless they receive HCC therapy resulting in a large AFP decrease.

A persistent problem is growth of the HCC during the months of waiting for a donor liver. HCCs of more than minimal size are typically treated with TACE/chemoembolization, radioembolization, or sorafenib in an attempt to stabilize the tumor during the wait for a donor liver. If the tumors grow beyond Milan criteria, the patient is typically withdrawn from the transplant eligibility list. Patients need to thus have regular, often 3-monthly scans and AFP measurements while on the liver transplant waiting list in order to detect HCC growth. A large clinical trial is currently in progress to assess whether adjuvant sorafenib therapy after liver transplant can reduce post-transplant recurrences. A small randomized trial has already shown some benefit for adjuvant sorafenib. Despite confidence in the radiological diagnosis of HCC without biopsy, it has recently been found that 20% of patients who supposedly had HCC did not have this diagnosis when the transplanted liver was examined pathologically. However, patients having HCC in a non-cirrhotic liver who are resected and then recur in the liver only, without presence of PVT, can be considered for "salvage" liver transplant. In addition, patients who have tumors outside Milan criteria can be "down-staged" with a tumor size and viability decrease using TACE/chemoembolization or radioembolization. In that case they may be re-considered for liver transplant. There is increasing use of live liver donors (a volunteer who has tissue compatibility and is willing to have part of the liver removed for organ donation), but the criteria for patients with HCC are the same as for non-living (cadaveric) donated livers.

Some patients have HCC recurrence after liver transplantation. If it is confined to the liver, then TACE/chemoembolization can be considered. If outside the liver, then sorafenib is likely to be used. The shortage of organs for all patients who might fit the Milan criteria, coupled with advances in safety of resection, especially for patients with a CP A cirrhosis score, has recently led to a re-evaluation of the benefits of resection for many patients who could be either transplanted or resected.

Summary for patients, families, and caregivers

People with small tumors and excellent liver function can potentially be cured of their HCC through ablation, surgical resection, and liver transplantation:

- Ablation is the killing or sterilizing of the cancerous cells in the liver. The cell killing works by applying concentrated radio waves (called radiofrequency ablation), extreme cold, extreme heat, or chemicals (alcohol) to the tumors. The most common method is radiofrequency ablation.

- Surgical resection means physically removing all of the cancerous tissue in the liver.
  - Surgeons can remove the cancerous parts of the liver because a healthy liver can regrow itself after removal of up to 70% of the original liver mass. However, a severely damaged (cirrhosis) liver cannot regrow. Thus, resection is not an option for patients with severe cirrhosis.
  - After a resection, the patient's HCC may come back in the 2–3 years after surgery. This is known as a recurrence. Researchers are studying how they can combine different therapies to stop recurrences from occurring after resection surgery.

- Liver transplantation is the surgical replacement of a patient's damaged liver by a donor's healthy liver. Liver transplantation is the only therapy with the potential to cure both the HCC and the underlying diseased liver at the same time. However, there are not many donor livers available. Also, while patients wait for an available liver, their cancer may get worse and preclude transplantation. Patients need to be monitored by scans and blood tests to keep an eye on their HCC and how it may be growing. Therefore, additional treatments might be given to slow down the tumor's growth while the patient waits for an available donor liver.

Further reading

1 Peng ZW, Zhang YJ, Chen MS, et al. Radiofrequency ablation with or without transcatheter arterial chemoembolization in the treatment of hepatocellular carcinoma: a prospective randomized trial. *J Clin Oncol*. 2013;31:426-432.

2 Sapisochin G, Castells L, Dopazo C, Bilbao I, Minguez B, Lázaro JL, Allende H, Balsells J, Caralt M, Charco R. Single HCC in cirrhotic patients: liver resection or liver transplantation? Long-term outcome according to an intention-to-treat basis. *Ann Surg Oncol*. 2013 Apr;20(4):1194-202.

3 Silva MF, Sapisochin G, Strasser SI, et al. Liver resection and transplantation offer similar 5-year survival for Child-Pugh-Turcotte A HCC-patients with a single nodule up to 5 cm: a multicenter, exploratory analysis. *Eur J Surg Oncol*. 2013;39:386-395.

4 Giannini EG, Savarino V, Farinati F, et al; Italian Liver Cancer (ITA.LI.CA) group. Influence of clinically significant portal hypertension on survival after hepatic resection for hepatocellular carcinoma in cirrhotic patients. *Liver Int*. 2013;33:1594-1600.

5 Tombesi P, Di Vece F, Sartori S. Resection vs thermal ablation of small hepatocellular carcinoma: What's the first choice? *World J Radiol*. 2013;5:1-4.

6 Hsu YC, Ho HJ, Wu MS, Lin JT, Wu CY. Postoperative peg-interferon plus ribavirin is associated with reduced recurrence of hepatitis C virus-related hepatocellular carcinoma. *Hepatology*. 2013;58:150-157.

7 Yin J, Li N, Han Y, Xue J, et al. Effect of antiviral treatment with nucleotide/nucleoside analogs on postoperative prognosis of hepatitis B virus-related hepatocellular carcinoma: a two-stage longitudinal clinical study. *J Clin Oncol*. 2013;31:4167.

8 Nault JC, De Reyniès A, Villanueva A, et al. A hepatocellular carcinoma 5-gene score associated with survival of patients after liver resection. *Gastroenterology*. 2013;145:176-187.

9 Iwatsuki S, Starzl TE, Sheahan DG, et al. Hepatic resection versus transplantation for hepatocellular carcinoma. *Ann Surg*. 1991;214:221-228.

10 Mazzaferro V, Regalia E, Doci R, et al. Liver transplantation for the treatment of small hepatocellular carcinomas in patients with cirrhosis. *N Engl J Med*. 1996;334:693-699.

11 Yao FY, Ferrell L, Bass NM, et al. Liver transplantation for hepatocellular carcinoma: expansion of the tumor size limits does not adversely impact survival. *Hepatology.* 2001;33:1394-1403.

12 Mazzaferro V, Llovet JM, Miceli R, et al; Metroticket Investigator Study Group Predicting survival after liver transplantation in patients with hepatocellular carcinoma beyond the Milan criteria: a retrospective, exploratory analysis. *Lancet Oncol.* 2009;10:35-43.

13 Clavien PA, Lesurtel M, Bossuyt PM, Gores GJ, Langer B, Perrier A; OLT for HCC Consensus Group. Recommendations for liver transplantation for hepatocellular carcinoma: an international consensus conference report. *Lancet Oncol.* 2012;13:e11-e22.

14 Cauchy F, Fuks D, Belghiti J. HCC: current surgical treatment concepts. *Langenbecks Arch Surg.* 2012;397:681-695.

15 Dhir M, Lyden ER, Smith LM, Are C. Comparison of outcomes of transplantation and resection in patients with early hepatocellular carcinoma: a meta-analysis. *HPB (Oxford).* 2012;14:635-645.

16 Carr BI. Hepatic artery chemoembolization for hepatocellular carcinoma recurrence confined to the transplanted liver. *Case Rep Oncol.* 2012;5:506-510.

Non-curative therapies (Group 2)

Hepatic artery chemotherapy, radioactive particle therapy and external beam radiotherapy

As previously mentioned, the liver receives its vascular supply via the portal vein and HCC receives its vascular supply via the hepatic artery. The ability to give high doses of chemotherapy to the HCC relatively selectively via injection through the skin into the hepatic artery, with considerable sparing of the underlying liver, has been the basis of most HCC therapy in recent decades for patients who cannot have surgery or ablation because of extensive hepatic tumor and who do not have extrahepatic metastases; this is called hepatic artery infusion (HAI) or transhepatic artery **chemoembolization (TACE)**. This can be a clinic or hospital procedure and is performed in the vascular radiology suite. A radiologist inserts a needle through the skin in the groin (upper leg area) and puts its tip into the femoral artery just underneath. A long plastic catheter is then inserted into the bore of the needle and threaded through the needle into the femoral artery and up into the aorta. This catheter tip is followed via a radiographic monitor and it is then threaded into the hepatic artery (similar to a cardiac angiogram). The radiologist then injects a dye to check which hepatic artery branch(es) feed the main HCC and threads the catheter into it/them, if possible. The chemotherapy is typically infused over 30–60 minutes. Often during this process, various particles are also injected to slow the blood flow into the artery (embolization). This has the dual effect of both permitting more drug to stay in the tumor area, rather than being washed into the rest of the liver by the blood flow, and it can also directly cause damage or necrosis to the tumor. The most frequently used drugs for the procedure are cisplatin or doxorubicin. The patient can either go home after several hours of observation, or after a hospital overnight stay for observation and safety monitoring. Analgesics and antiemetics (antinauseants) are also administered before and during the TACE/chemoembolization procedure. The chemotherapy is designed to kill the cancer cells and usually has little effect on the rest of a normal liver, especially if it is infused into a hepatic artery branch. It can be potentially dangerous to patients with CP C cirrhosis, with any elevation of blood bilirubin levels >2.0 mg/dl, or with more than minimal ascites (fluid in the abdomen from cirrhosis). It seems to be fairly safe in the presence of single PVT if that is unilateral, but not if it is bilateral or involving the main portal vein trunk. The TACE/chemoembolization procedure is typically repeated each 3 to 6 months, depending on follow-up scans of the liver and its tumors. If the tumor is stable, then less frequent treatments are better due to liver safety. It is widely used for multifocal or extensive or large HCCs, but has little value if distant metastases are present (see sorafenib section below on page 37). Recently, doxorubicin-containing drug-eluting beads have been introduced for this purpose and have been shown to be safe and may produce longer tumor responses, but definitive trials are awaited. Despite use of TACE/chemoembolization for more than 30 years, there is no clear evidence which of several chemotherapy agents is best. Although doxorubicin and cisplatin are popular, there are no comparative data. In this author's opinion, cisplatin may be superior. A mixture of doxorubicin, mitomycin C, and cisplatin at low doses compared to any of the component drugs alone is popular, but this has not yet been supported by comparative clinical trial evidence. Similarly, many agents or particles have been used for the embolization, but without comparative studies, the choice is usually based on the radiologist's preference.

Locoregional therapy using radioactive spheres (glass-based TheraSphere® Yttrium-90 Microspheres [Nordion Inc. for BTG International, Ottawa, Canada] or resin-based SIR-Spheres® microspheres [SIRTeX Corp, North Sydney, Australia]) have been introduced into clinical use for several years. TheraSphere has have US Food and Drug Administration (FDA) approval for HCC as a part of a humanitarian device exemption rule of the FDA for compassionate use for new agents for rare diseases. SIR-Spheres has pre-market approval for metastatic colorectal cancer. Both agents are currently in clinical trials for HCC, and patients can often receive these promising therapies through compassionate approval by local hospital ethics committees (eg, institutional review boards), even without participating in a clinical trial.

The spheres are 20–30 microns in diameter (less than a human hair or 3-fold the size of a red blood cell) and carry radioactivity from the beta particle-emitting isotope [90]Yttrium. As the isotope has a 64-hour half-life (ie, has lost half its radioactivity in 3 days and has minimal radioactivity after 10 days) and a typical radioactive tissue penetration of 2.5 mm (maximum 1 cm), neither family nor medical staff will be exposed to its radiation after it has been injected. Several studies have shown its safety, but there have not yet been any completed randomized trials to mark a gold standard for this therapy. Nevertheless, whereas TACE/chemoembolization is dangerous in the presence of complete PVT and needs to be performed with great caution in the presence of the major branch PVT, the use of radioactive spheres appears safe in this setting for the treatment of HCC confined to the liver, and in the presence of any PVT. Responses have been reported for 35–50% of patients using either TACE/chemoembolization or radioembolization, with average survival of 12 to 18 months for these unresectable patients, depending on their liver function. Comparison trials with radioactive spheres and TACE/chemoembolization or with sorafenib are in progress.

Although the term radioembolization has been used, this is technically true for only SIR-Spheres. While both TheraSphere and SIR-Spheres use [90]Yttrium labeled spheres, they are not identical products. TheraSphere is a pure radiation treatment, with much higher doses of radiation and lower number of spheres being delivered than SIR-Spheres. By contrast, SIR-Spheres have lower radiation, but a much higher sphere number per dose, giving an embolization effect (like TACE/chemoembolization) in addition to its radiation, which TheraSphere does not. The ideal product likely has more spheres than TheraSphere and more radioactivity than SIR-Spheres. TheraSphere is approved for HCC therapy only as a humanitarian device exemption product by FDA. SIR-Spheres is approved, but only for colon cancer metastases, so far.

[131]I-Lipiodol is a radioisotope available in Japan, but not in the USA. It seems attractive due to its minor toxicities and is the only agent so far tested that has been shown to improve recurrence-free survival after surgical resection.

External beam radiotherapy has not generally been employed for the liver, due to hepatotoxicity. More finely focused radiation beams, as in intensity-modulated radiation therapy or high intensity image modulated radiation therapy (stereotactic body radiation therapy), appear to be less toxic. External beam therapy has been used in several Japanese reports for treatment of main stem or main branch PVT. Proton beam therapy is another new approach that is in process of validation.

Summary for patients, families, and caregivers

Anticancer drugs called chemotherapy can be used to treat patients with multiple or large tumors in the liver. Chemotherapy is injected directly into the liver artery, which feeds the HCC, called the hepatic artery. The injection process is called transhepatic artery chemoembolization (TACE). Since the chemotherapy is injected into the tumor, the rest of the liver is relatively safe from the toxic effects of the treatment. This is possible because the non-tumor liver mostly receives its blood supply by another blood vessel (the hepatic portal vein), so normal liver cells should not be affected.

The chemotherapy is injected by inserting a needle through the skin of the upper leg area (groin) and into the underlying artery, and then a small flexible tube (a catheter) is inserted into the needle to reach the HCC. A radiologist injects a dye to find where the tumors are in the liver. If possible, the radiologist will put the catheter directly into the arteries feeding the tumors. The catheter will then deliver the chemotherapy to the tumor(s). The treatment is usually given over 30–60 minutes and repeated every 3–6 months. Two commonly used chemotherapy drugs are cisplatin or doxorubicin. Other drugs are given during the procedure to prevent side effects of the chemotherapy. Side effects include pain, nausea, diarrhea, and fatigue. After the session is finished, the healthcare team monitors the patient for a few hours or overnight to make sure they are safe.

A similar treatment to chemotherapy involves the infusion of radioactive beads into the artery feeding the HCC (radioembolization). Another treatment called external beam radiotherapy is not commonly used, as this treatment may destroy normal cells as well as cancerous cells unless it is focused very accurately.

Further reading

1   Kulik LM, Carr BI, Mulcahy MF, et al. Safety and efficacy of 90Y radiotherapy for hepatocellular carcinoma with and without portal vein thrombosis. *Hepatology*. 2008;47:71-81.

2   Carr BI, Kondragunta V, Buch SC, Branch RA. Therapeutic equivalence in survival for hepatic arterial chemoembolization and yttrium 90 microsphere treatments in unresectable hepatocellular carcinoma: a two-cohort study. *Cancer*. 2010;116:1305-1314.

3   Kudo M, Izumi N, Kokudo N, et al; HCC Expert Panel of Japan Society of Hepatology. Management of hepatocellular carcinoma in Japan: Consensus-Based Clinical Practice Guidelines proposed by the Japan Society of Hepatology (JSH) 2010 updated version. *Dig Dis*. 2011;29:339-364.

4   de Lope CR, Tremosini S, Forner A, Reig M, Bruix J. Management of HCC. *J Hepatol*. 2012;56 Suppl 1:S75-S87.

5   Cammá C, Schepis F, Orlando A, et al. Transarterial chemoembolization for unresectable hepatocellular carcinoma: meta-analysis of randomized controlled trials. *Radiology*. 2002;224:47-54.

6   Kudo M. Treatment of Advanced Hepatocellular Carcinoma with Emphasis on Hepatic Arterial Infusion Chemotherapy and Molecular Targeted Therapy. *Liver Cancer*. 2012;1:62-70.

7   Burrel M, Reig M, Forner A, et al. Survival of patients with hepatocellular carcinoma treated by transarterial chemoembolisation (TACE) using Drug Eluting Beads. Implications for clinical practice and trial design. *J Hepatol*. 2012;56:1330-1335.

8   Lo CM, Ngan H, Tso WK, et al. Randomized controlled trial of transarterial lipiodol chemoembolization for unresectable hepatocellular carcinoma. *Hepatology*. 2002;35:1164-1171.

9   Llovet JM1, Real MI, Montaña X, et al; Barcelona Liver Cancer Group. Arterial embolisation or chemoembolisation versus symptomatic treatment in patients with unresectable hepatocellular carcinoma: a randomised controlled trial. *Lancet*. 2002;359:1734-1739.

Systemic drugs (Group 2)

Systemic chemotherapy

Many reports and clinical trials have been documented over several decades on systemic or intravenous administration of a large number of different chemotherapeutic agents. Their effect on tumor shrinkage is small and inconsistent, toxicity can be high, and there is no proven survival advantage so far reported.

Hormones and non-cytotoxic agents

Several hormones and male and female hormone-manipulating agents have been assessed in recent years, including tamoxifen, leuprolide, megestrol, sandostatin, and the immune modulating agents interferon and thalidomide. Although they do not have the toxicities of chemotherapy, none of them have been shown to extend survival compared to no treatment; thus, they have all been generally abandoned for treatment of HCC. This is similarly true for interferon and arsenic trioxide.

Multikinase inhibitors

In the last three decades, research has made great progress in the identification of several key biochemical pathways that are involved in cancer growth, especially regarding cell growth and the new tumor blood vessels (angiogenesis) that appear necessary for most cancer types to grow beyond a minimal size. The enzymes associated with many of the steps of these pathways have been identified, purified, and either antibodies or specific chemical inhibitors have been made against them or against their cellular target molecules (often cell surface receptors). The result has been a huge increase in new therapeutic agents being investigated in clinical trials for the treatment of a range of cancers including HCC. The remarkable thing is that this approach represents a paradigm shift away from (largely nonspecific) cell poisons or cytotoxins (chemotherapy), but instead to agents that work by modifying tumor cell behavior in various ways, either by directly inhibiting crucial steps in the cell growth pathway(s) or by antagonizing steps in supportive activities, such as angiogenesis, cell differentiation, cell adhesion, migration (metastasis) or immune modulation. Furthermore, because the major mechanisms by which this new set of agents (drugs and antibodies) work is often understood, for the first time in cancer therapy, predictive chemical or molecular tests can be developed to determine which patient's cancer cells have the necessary biochemical configuration or gene expression profile to be able to respond to these new therapies (ie, personalized medicine). If they do not, then both time and money need not be wasted in futile therapy for several months as might be the case with chemotherapy.

Sorafenib

The first systemic agent that was successful in Phase III randomized, clinical trial evaluation was sorafenib (NEXAVAR), a multikinase inhibitor. Kinases are enzymes that phosphorylate and thereby usually activate other proteins. Sorafenib can be taken orally (tablet), unlike most chemotherapy, and is the first agent of any kind to be approved by the FDA for therapy of advanced or surgically untreatable (and un-ablatable) HCC because it showed a survival advantage in treated patients. Two Phase III multicenter, randomized, double-blind, placebo-controlled trials showed that patients with HCC treated with sorafenib had longer survival than patients with HCC who did not receive any treatment. SHARP (Sorafenib HCC Assessment Randomized Protocol Trial) Investigators found the median overall survival was 10.7 versus 7.9 months when patients were given either sorafenib (400 mg twice daily) or placebo, respectively. A similar study in patients treated with the same dose of sorafenib and placebo in Asia–Pacific populations (specifically China, South Korea, and Taiwan) found the medial overall survival to be 6.5 versus 4.2 months, respectively. There was a decrease in the tumor vascularity, which is a hallmark of tumor cell viability, on the patients' radiology scans. This has two major consequences for HCC oncology. First, since the vascularity decreases, usually without total tumor size decrease, radiology scans need to be optimized to find some way of measuring (quantitating) the vascular changes. Second, it forces us to re-evaluate the significance of tumor response in clinical oncology (see response section, below). In the chemotherapy era, it was generally accepted that only a drug that shrinks tumors is useful, but results from sorafenib clinical trials have shown that this idea may need to be finessed. Furthermore, it was also generally thought that the stability of tumor size (neither growing nor shrinking) likely represented a therapy failure. However, the sorafenib data are supporting the idea that stable disease might also be desirable (ie, if the cancer does not grow, it will not kill you). Thus, in addition to having a survival benefit, sorafenib has helped us learn more about this cancer.

Despite this step forward, there are some concerns. There was a modest increase of 10 weeks in survival in the sorafenib group compared to the placebo group, and oddly there was minimal tumor shrinkage (2% partial responses; see the discussion on responses to therapy, below). Because the tumor masses did not shrink, the tumors were still mostly present and eventually were able to regrow. There are also considerable toxicities, including a profound tiredness and weakness, in about 30% of patients that can result in cessation of therapy, patient refusal to continue or, most frequently, a temporary discontinuation and restart of therapy at a lower dose. Diarrhea and hand–foot syndrome toxicity occurred in about 10% of patients. Hand–foot syndrome is redness, swelling, and painful blisters on the palms of the hands and soles of the feet, the latter making walking difficult for patients. The role of sorafenib seems to be mainly for the treatment of patients with HCC metastases outside the liver or after first-line therapy with TACE/chemoembolization or radioembolization has failed. It is also used as first-line therapy in the presence of PVT (so is radioembolization). Clinical trials are ongoing in a variety of circumstances, such as bridge to transplantation (during the wait for a donor organ), in combination with TACE/chemoembolization or radioembolization, and as an adjuvant to prevent recurrences after resection or ablation. In contrast to TACE/chemoembolization, sorafenib demonstrated a favorable safety profile in patients with CP B cirrhosis.

Other multikinase inhibitors

The success of sorafenib has given optimism for many other agents that inhibit similar or parallel pathways. Some, such as sunitinib, brivanib, linifanib, and bevacizumab, have disappointed in recent major clinical trials, but many new agents are currently being tested. These trials can possibly lead to combination therapies with sorafenib to improve upon its actions, or new therapies may be available for patients whose tumors grow after sorafenib treatment. One candidate for this is fluoro-sorafenib or regorafenib (STIVARGA® [Bayer HealthCare Pharmaceuticals Inc., Wayne, NJ]) a close analog of sorafenib, which is currently in clinical trials. Regorafenib is approved for the second-line treatment of colorectal cancer metastases and ongoing clinical studies are assessing the safety and efficacy of this agent in patients with HCC. Other promising candidates include several inhibitors of epidermal growth factor receptor and fibroblast growth factor receptors, which mediate the actions of two natural HCC growth-stimulating chemicals in the body, epidermal growth factor and fibroblast growth factor, respectively, as well as inhibitors of the Met receptor (tivantinib also known as ARQ 197).

New approaches with kinase inhibitors

The model for combining drugs came initially from tuberculosis and other antimicrobial therapies followed by cancer chemotherapy. The idea was that drugs with different modes of action and/or with different toxicity profiles might be combined to produce better bacterial or cancer cell kill, or to decrease the likelihood of emerging drug resistance. Thus, several trials are now ongoing, which combine sorafenib with other newer kinase inhibitors. Although several new therapies have not been successful in showing equality or superiority with less toxicity to sorafenib, they may yet have therapeutic usefulness, as none of them have effects on the identical mix of cell targets or to the same degree. Furthermore, since TACE/chemoembolization and radioembolization can shrink tumors whereas sorafenib extends survival but does not shrink tumors appreciably, several trials are ongoing to combine the modalities (eg, sorafenib plus TACE/chemoembolization or sorafenib plus radioembolization versus either alone). Many practitioners are already combining sorafenib plus TACE/chemoembolization until the data to support it are available from ongoing trials.

There are no data yet to support any particular therapy in patients who have failed sorafenib; enrolling the patient in a clinical trial may be the best option for this situation. However, if a patient has not been treated with TACE/chemoembolization or radioembolization, then either option could be considered if they do not have metastatic disease or main-stem PVT. As previously mentioned, RFA is often combined with TACE/chemoembolization for tumors ≥5 cm or with satellite lesions; however, RFA followed by sorafenib might also be a reasonable approach for larger lesions >3 cm or several lesions >1 and <5 nodules. In the presence of main trunk PVT, only sorafenib or radioembolization are currently considered to be safe.

Summary for patients, families, and caregivers

Systemic drugs are medications that travel through the patient's bloodstream and can affect the patient's whole body. Unlike the treatment of many other cancers, injecting anticancer drugs directly into the patient's bloodstream (systemic chemotherapy) has not been very successful in treating HCC. It is associated with side effects that limit its use and has limited effectiveness.

However, new therapies are making big advances for patients and their treatment. New oral medications change a cancer cell's behavior by preventing important steps in the tumor's growth process. One example of such a drug is sorafenib. Sorafenib is the first drug approved for patients with advanced HCC who cannot have surgery or ablation. The aim of sorafenib treatment is to try to stop or slow down the tumor's growth and slow down the growth of new blood vessels within the tumor. Common side effects of sorafenib include tiredness, weakness, diarrhea, and painful redness, swelling, and blisters on the palms of the hands and feet (called hand–foot syndrome).

There are other drugs that work in a similar or complementary way to sorafenib. Research is being done to see if these drugs can be used with each other or with other treatments for HCC.

Further reading

1 Bruix J, Raoul JL, Sherman M, et al. Efficacy and safety of sorafenib in patients with advanced hepatocellular carcinoma: subanalyses of a phase III trial. *J Hepatol.* 2012;57:821-829.

2 Zhang T, Ding X, Wei D, et al. Sorafenib improves the survival of patients with advanced hepatocellular carcinoma: a meta-analysis of randomized trials. *Anticancer Drugs.* 2010;21:326-332.

3 Villanueva A, Llovet JM. Targeted therapies for hepatocellular carcinoma. *Gastroenterology.* 2011;140:1410-1426.

4 Wei Z, Doria C, Liu Y. Targeted therapies in the treatment of advanced hepatocellular carcinoma. *Clin Med Insights Oncol.* 2013;7:87-102.

5 Tanaka S, Arii S. Molecular targeted therapies in hepatocellular carcinoma. *Semin Oncol.* 2012;39:486-492.

6 Llovet JM, Ricci S, Mazzaferro V, et al; SHARP Investigators Study Group. Sorafenib in advanced hepatocellular carcinoma. *N Engl J Med.* 2008;359:378-390.

7 Cheng AL, Kang YK, Chen Z, et al. Efficacy and safety of sorafenib in patients in the Asia-Pacific region with advanced hepatocellular carcinoma: a phase III randomised, double-blind, placebo-controlled trial. *Lancet Oncol.* 2009;10:25-34.

8 Kim HY, Park JW. Molecularly targeted therapies for hepatocellular carcinoma: sorafenib as a stepping stone. *Dig Dis.* 2011;29:303-309.

9 Zhu AX. Molecularly targeted therapy for advanced hepatocellular carcinoma in 2012: current status and future perspectives. *Semin Oncol.* 2012;39:493-502.

Assessment of responses to therapy: what do tumor size responses signify?

The radiological measurement of tumor size and number has been an important patient management tool since the introduction of chemotherapy for cancer therapy. A diminution in tumor size and number has signified a desired treatment outcome (Figure 6), and an enlargement of size or increase in number of nodules is generally not encouraging and implies a failure of treatment. Meanwhile, stable disease has been considered unsatisfactory, neither good nor bad. It has always been understood that survival time is the gold standard for assessing treatment effectiveness, whether this is within the context of a clinical trial or not. Since survival time can take months or years to determine, a tumor response has been thought to be a clinically useful surrogate, and especially useful in an individual patient since the treating physician has to determine whether to discontinue an ineffective therapy or continue it in the absence of progression (increase in size or number of tumor nodules). Several accepted response classification schemes have been used, including schemes from the World Health Organization (WHO) and response evaluation criteria in solid tumors (RECIST), the latter recently modified (mRECIST) to include an assessment of tumor vascularity changes. Assessments have included: complete response or disappearance of tumor; partial response or shrinkage of tumor; stable disease; progressive disease or growth in tumor size or number. The mRECIST is particularly useful for HCC, as it is a highly vascular cancer and a lessening of tumor vascularity on CT or MRI scan is a measure of decreased tumor viability or of increased cell death (necrosis) (Figure 7). Furthermore, for the 50% of patients with HCC who have elevated blood AFP levels, a consistent change in level is a quite reliable marker for tumor response or failure of response to the therapy.

It is generally accepted that an increase in tumor size or number indicates a therapy failure. But, it has also long been clear that there is a poor relationship between tumor response/shrinkage and survival. For example, fast-growing solid tumors, such as ovarian and small-cell lung cancer, can quickly respond to chemotherapy by tumor shrinkage, but the responses often do not hold, as the tumor develops resistance to chemotherapy and can then re-grow. By contrast, in the sorafenib SHARP trial only 2% of patients had tumor size shrinkage in the treatment group, yet there was an increase in median survival in treated compared to placebo patients. Thus, there seems to be an uncoupling between response and survival. Furthermore, 70% of the treated group had stable disease. Perhaps this explains the issue, since multikinase inhibitors interfere with tumor growth as they were designed to do, but may not actually kill the tumors, as cytotoxic chemotherapy was designed to do. This concept provides a rationale for combining sorafenib with TACE/chemoembolization or radioembolization, and that perhaps "stable disease" is a desirable outcome in its own right for therapies that are not curative, such as TACE/chemoembolization, radioembolization or sorafenib. Stable disease means that the HCC is not growing, which may be a desirable goal if future studies show that this therapeutic result relates to enhanced survival.

Summary for patients, families, and caregivers

Sorafenib and similar therapies in development can slow tumor growth. By slowing the tumor's growth, some patients have longer survival. This means that patients can live longer even though the sorafenib did not kill or shrink all of their tumors. Generally, healthcare professionals have focused on shrinking or killing the cancer, rather than preventing cancer growth. This means that healthcare professionals may have to re-focus on slowing or stopping the cancer from growing – rather than focusing on shrinking and killing the cancer – in order to help their patients live longer, which is the main aim of HCC therapy.

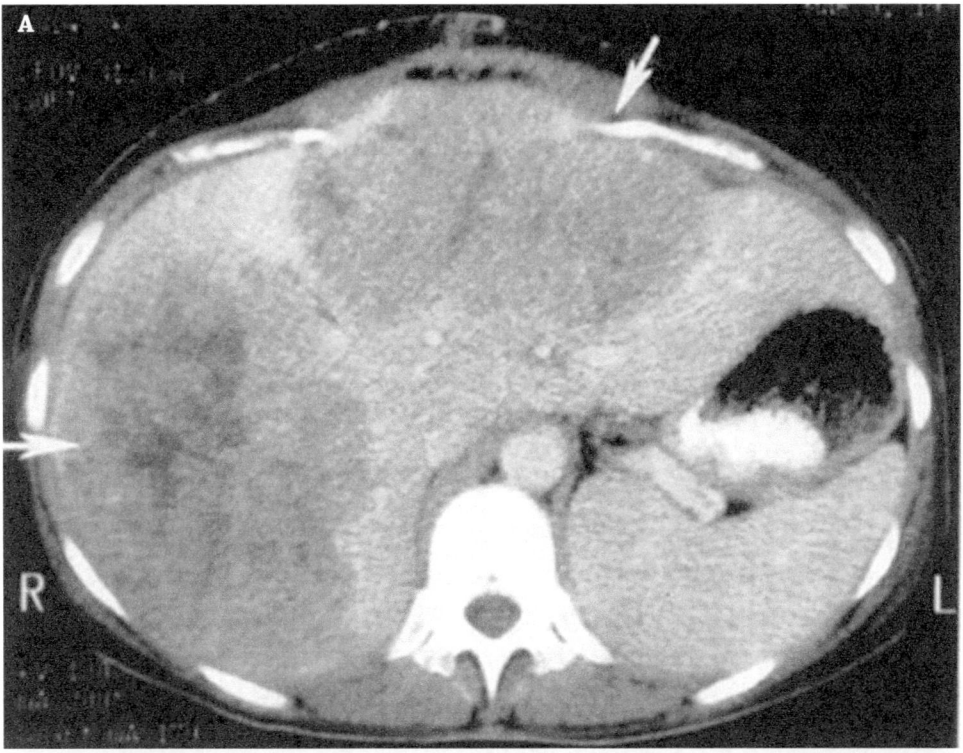

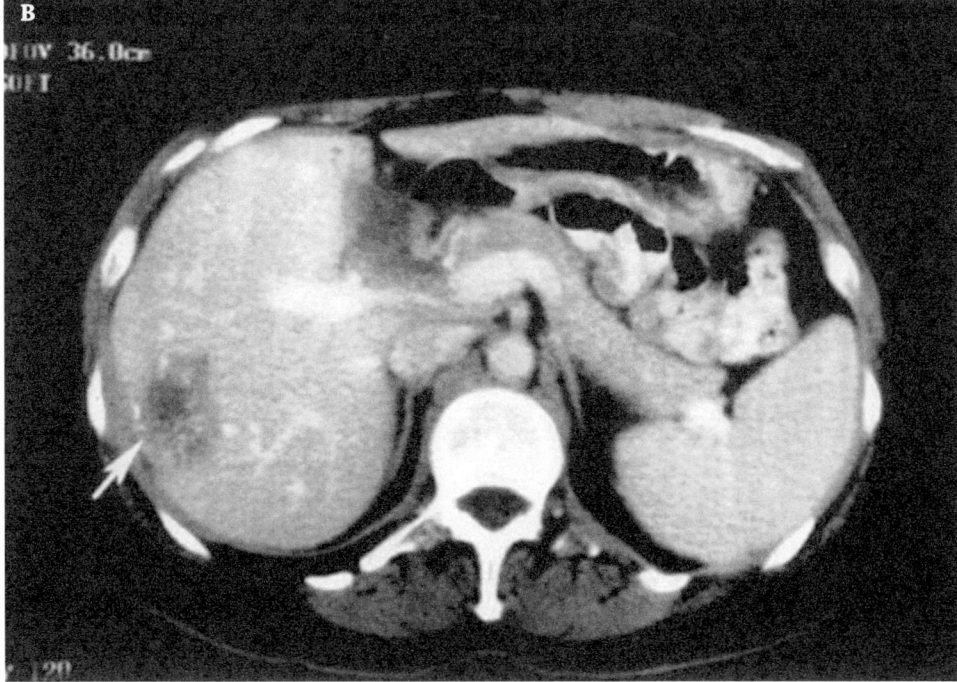

Figure 6 Types of hepatocellular carcinoma size response to therapy.
A, pre-chemotherapy, anterior spine; **B,** post-chemotherapy, anterior spine.

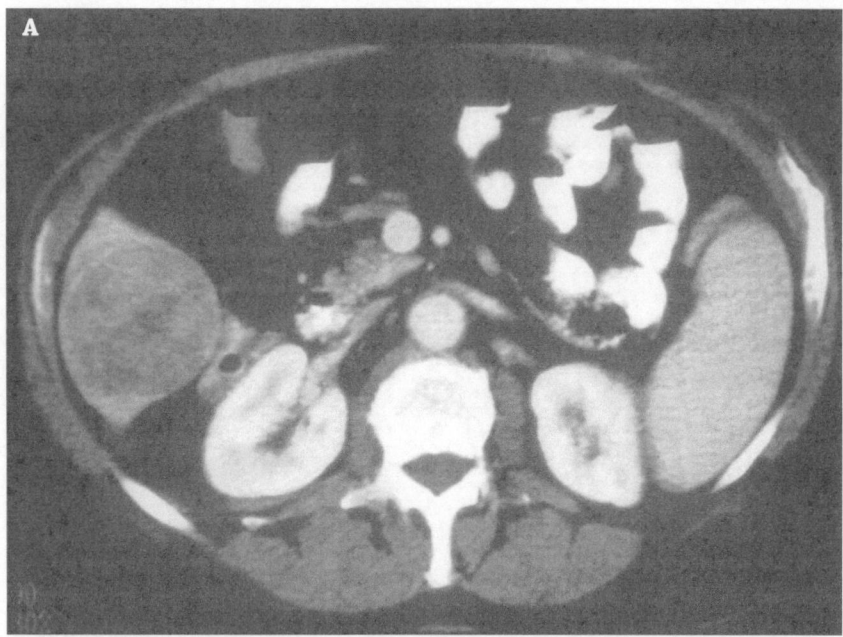

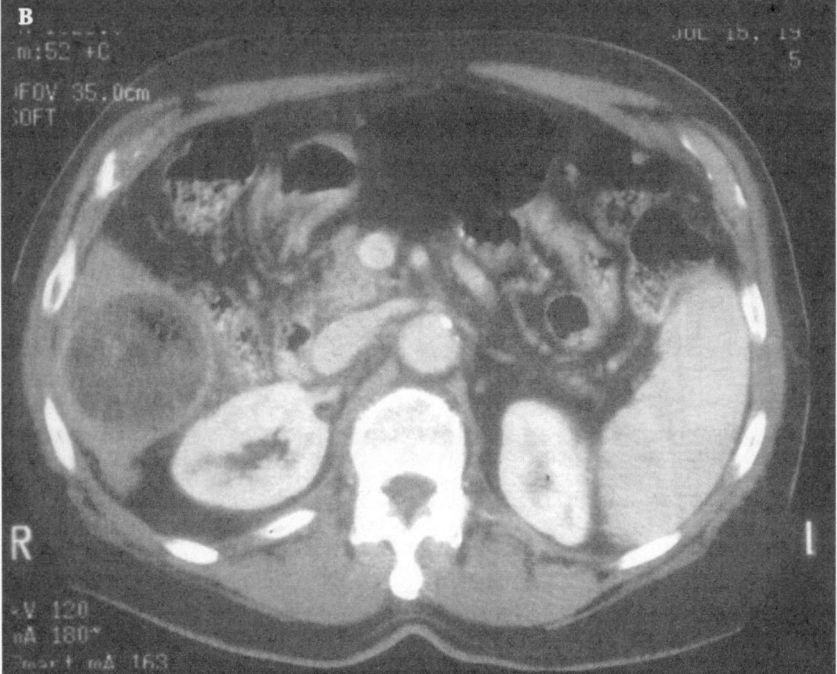

Figure 7 CAT scan showing vascular response to therapy without change in tumor size. Reproduced with permission from © Springer Science+Business Media, 2014; Carr BI. *Hepatocellular Carcinoma.* 2nd ed. New York, NY: Springer Science+Business Media; 2010.

Further reading

1 Riaz A, Ryu RK, Kulik LM, et al. Alpha-fetoprotein response after locoregional therapy for hepatocellular carcinoma: oncologic marker of radiologic response, progression, and survival. *J Clin Oncol.* 2009;27:5734-5742.

2 Llovet JM, Ricci S, Mazzaferro V, et al; SHARP Investigators Study Group. Sorafenib in advanced hepatocellular carcinoma. *N Engl J Med.* 2008;359:378-390.

Hepatitis therapy is also anticancer therapy

Considerations of hepatitis therapy play a role in three aspects of HCC management:

1. Prevention. Hepatitis B (HBV) prevention by HBV vaccination, or avoidance of hepatitis C (HCV) contamination of blood bank supplies, both to prevent HCC development.
2. Antiviral treatment of patients who already have HBV and HCV to prevent HCC.
3. Antiviral treatment of patients with resected HCC who have HBV or HCV to prevent HCC recurrence.

As discussed earlier, HCC seems to arise in most cases (approximately 85%) from necro-inflammatory liver disease (typically by cirrhosis) caused most often by HBV, HCV, alcoholism, food contamination by aflatoxin B_1, obesity, or a combination of any of these predisposing factors. The greatest contributor worldwide is HBV, which is particularly common in patients with HCC in Asia. Most HBV is transmitted by the mother to her fetus in the blood stream as the placental membrane of the baby breaks during birth. Due to a massive neonatal HBV vaccination program in Asia (and more recently in the West), the last two decades have seen a remarkable decrease in childhood and adolescent HBV rates. The early signs of an expected resultant decrease in HCC have already appeared in China and Taiwan. This HBV prevention program will have enormous effects in decreasing Asian HCC in the coming decades. However, in Japan, where HCV infection typically originates from past HCV-contaminated blood transfusions, an expected decrease will come with a change in modern blood bank screening methods.

There are millions of adults who are long-time HBV carriers and for whom HBV vaccination and thus prevention will not help. Nevertheless, recent advances in effective HBV therapy are beginning to show that successful treatment of patients with chronic HBV infection will translate into a decrease in subsequent HCC incidence. New anti-HCV therapies offer similar grounds for optimism.

The high HCC recurrence rates after HCC resection has led to many studies of anticancer therapy after treatment to prevent growth of presumptive microscopic metastases that cannot be seen by the surgeon or on radiology scans. To date, most of these adjuvant trials have been ineffective. Despite this, recent trials of HBV and HCV therapy post-resection have shown that antiviral therapy can decrease the rates of HCC recurrence post-resection (this may likely also apply to ablation). This suggests that either the growth of microscopic to macroscopic recurrences are influenced by the hepatitis-mediated inflammation (see microenvironment section), or that the recurrences are not really recurrences, but actually new HCCs formed from cirrhotic nodules (throughout the liver) under the continuing influence of viral factors or virus-mediated inflammation.

Thus, all three approaches involve antivirus hepatitis therapies as being important aspects of HCC prevention, suppression, or minimization of recurrence.

Summary for patients, families, and caregivers

Hepatitis B and C infection are two major causes of HCC. If hepatitis can be prevented by vaccines or managed by antiviral therapy, then HCC may be prevented or managed as well. HCC can be managed by hepatitis therapy in three ways:

1. Vaccination – Hepatitis B infection can be prevented by hepatitis B vaccinations. Thus, hepatitis B vaccinations can prevent HCC too. This has been proven by a large scale neonatal hepatitis B vaccination program in Asia where rates of HCC have started to decrease. Hepatitis C can be prevented by screening blood bank supplies or use of sterile needles for injection of medicines by medical personnel or of drugs by addicts.
2. Hepatitis therapy – Hepatitis therapies can decrease the likelihood of chronic hepatitis infection from turning into HCC.
3. Hepatitis therapy after surgery – A patient with hepatitis can develop new HCC even after they have undergone surgery to remove the cancer. The patient should keep receiving hepatitis therapies after surgery to reduce the chances of developing HCC again.

Further reading

1 McMahon BJ, Bulkow LR, Singleton RJ, et al. Elimination of hepatocellular carcinoma and acute hepatitis B in children 25 years after a hepatitis B newborn and catch-up immunization program. *Hepatology*. 2011;54:801-807.

2 Ni YH, Chen DS. Hepatitis B vaccination in children: the Taiwan experience. *Pathol Biol (Paris)*. 2010;58:296-300.

3 Chang MH. Prevention of hepatitis B virus infection and liver cancer. *Recent Results Cancer Res*. 2014;193:75-95.

4 Hosaka T, Suzuki F, Kobayashi M, et al. Long-term entecavir treatment reduces hepatocellular carcinoma incidence in patients with hepatitis B virus infection. *Hepatology*. 2013;58:98-107.

5 Urata Y, Kubo S, Takemura S, et al. Effects of antiviral therapy on long-term outcome after liver resection for hepatitis B virus-related hepatocellular carcinoma. *J Hepatobiliary Pancreat Sci*. 2012;19:685-696.

6 Lok AS. Does antiviral therapy for hepatitis B and C prevent hepatocellular carcinoma? *J Gastroenterol Hepatol*. 2011;26:221-227.

7 Yin J, Li N, Han Y, et al. Effect of antiviral treatment with nucleotide/nucleoside analogs on postoperative prognosis of hepatitis B virus-related hepatocellular carcinoma: a two-stage longitudinal clinical study. *J Clin Oncol*. 2013;31:3647-3655.

8 Huang LM, Lu CY, Chen DS. Hepatitis B virus infection, its sequelae, and prevention by vaccination. *Curr Opin Immunol*. 2011;23:237-243.

Section 4

The whole patient setting

Therapy decisions for the individual patient: importance of a **multidisciplinary team approach**

The previous radiology and therapy sections show that many specialties are involved in the care, support, decision making, and management of any individual patient with hepatocellular carcinoma (HCC). The specialists include the gastroenterologist/hepatologist, diagnostic radiologist, interventional radiologist, pathologist, oncologist, nuclear medicine professional (radiation safety and radiation pharmacy for radioembolization), liver surgeon, liver transplant surgeon, chemotherapy nurse, and data/IT manager as well as a social worker, a psychologist, and often a dietitian. In practice, all of these professionals need to be involved in the direct care of the patient (except IT) at some phase in the disease process, but especially to discuss the individual patient together after the initial diagnostic work up and for treatment planning. The complexity of the two diseases usually requires more than the skills of a single practitioner. In addition, for many treatment decisions, more than one choice is available at any time in the disease progression, and the strength of the evidence for each approach can be variable and the approach can also depend on the local physician's skills or experience (eg, resection, radiofrequency ablation [RFA], percutaneous ethanol injection, cryoablation, or transarterial chemoembolization [TACE] versus radioembolization). Thus, the best advice and service available to any individual patient may require cross-specialty discussions that are often available mainly in large medical centers. Geography may impose some limitations on patients' ability to receive this care, but the multispecialty team is the optimal management choice for patient care and treating HCC .

Summary for patients, families, and caregivers

More than one healthcare professional is needed to care for patients with HCC. A multidisciplinary team of specialist physicians, nurses, and other healthcare professionals is required to ensure that their patients receive the best possible medical care. The healthcare team's different backgrounds and knowledge will help support the patient and manage their HCC and liver diseases. The specialists include:

- Gastroenterologist – a physician who manages the digestive system (stomach, colon, intestines, etc)
- Hepatologist – a physician who manages the liver and related organs (gallbladder, pancreas, etc)
- Radiologists – a physician who uses images to diagnose and treat diseases
- Pathologist – a physician who studies and diagnoses diseases
- Oncologist – a physician who manages cancers and administers anticancer medicines
- Nuclear medicine professional – a healthcare professional who studies and manages the use of radiation and nuclear medicine for imagining and related treatments
- Liver surgeon, liver transplant surgeon – physicians who perform surgeries related to the liver and transplanting the liver
- Chemotherapy nurse – a nurse who administers anticancer drugs (chemotherapy) and supports the patients during treatment

Continues over

B. I. Carr, *Understanding Liver Cancer*, DOI: 10.1007/978-1-910315-02-6_4,
© Springer Healthcare 2014

Summary for patients, families, and caregivers (continued)

- Dieticians – healthcare professionals who advise patients on healthy eating
- Psychologists – healthcare professionals who evaluate, diagnose, and treat patients' mental processes and behaviors
- Social workers – professionals who help patients improve their quality of life and well-being

Psychosocial considerations, family, support groups

Most patients with any type of cancer do not live in isolation, but as part of a context that involves a partner, family, community, or all three. Not only does a deadly disease have an effect on family and dependents, but people close to the patient can often play a crucial role in patient coping and compliance with medical advice. While obvious, this has particular relevance to HCC in several respects. First, the liver transplant team normally requires functional family support for the patient to endure the treatment-associated procedures and symptoms as well as to comply with treatment recommendations. Second, in many ways, HCC is a psychosocial disease. This is particularly true of HCC induced by chronic alcoholism or recreational drug use and any associated hepatitis infection; these two factors often coexist in the same patient. Furthermore, alcoholism (and cigarette smoking) can increase the risks of HCC in patients with aflatoxin B_1 exposure, as well as in patients who are hepatitis carriers. In addition to these self-inflicted behavioral issues, many patients developed HCV as a result of contaminated blood transfusions before there were tests for HCV. Thus, considerations of guilt, remorse, or victimization add to the general psychological issues of patients with HCC who have the same fears and hopes that are common to most patients with cancer. Men seem to have more difficulty than women in sharing and expressing their fears and anger. The sharing of their emotions can lead to support from friends, family, or cancer support groups. All these considerations are important factors in the treatment of the patient with HCC and are often necessary in helping patients cope and comply with treatment recommendations, as well as coping with the side effects of hepatitis and cancer therapies. The whole panoply of psychosocial support is increasingly accepted as a standard and necessary aspect of good patient management.

Summary for patients, families, and caregivers

A diagnosis of HCC can affect the psychological well-being of the affected person as well as their partner, family, friends, and other caregivers. Patients may feel guilty, remorseful, or victimized after a diagnosis because risk factors of HCC are sometimes preventable (like drug abuse, alcoholism, and infection from a blood transfusion). An individual's social support system can play an important role in coming to terms with the disease and taking their treatment as instructed.

Further reading

1   Carr BI, Steel J. *Psychological Aspects of Cancer.* New York, NY: Springer Science+Business Media; 2013.

2   Carr BI, Pujol L. Pain at presentation and survival in hepatocellular carcinoma. *J Pain.* 2010;11:988-993.

3   Steel J, Baum A, Carr B. Quality of life in patients diagnosed with primary hepatocellular carcinoma: hepatic arterial infusion of Cisplatin versus 90-Yttrium microspheres (Therasphere). *Psychooncology.* 2004;13:73-79.

4   Steel JL, Geller DA, Gamblin TC, Olek MC, Carr BI. Depression, immunity, and survival in patients with hepatobiliary carcinoma. *J Clin Oncol.* 2007;25:2397-2405.

5   Davila JA, Duan Z, McGlynn KA, El-Serag HB. Utilization and outcomes of palliative therapy for hepatocellular carcinoma: a population-based study in the United States. *J Clin Gastroenterol.* 2012;46:71-77.

Section 5

New directions

A series of both scientific and clinical advances is changing the management of hepatocellular carcinoma (HCC). These include:

1. The identification of preventable and treatable causal factors, including hepatitis B (HBV), hepatitis C (HCV), alcoholism, and obesity (non-alcoholic steatotic hepatitis [NASH]).

2. The characterization of molecular and proteomic profiles for HCC prognosis, disease subtyping, and rational drug selection.

3. The identification of circulating tumor cells for non-invasive molecular typing.

4. The identification of tumor stem/progenitor cell characteristics for HCC subtyping and as treatment targets.

5. The development of large numbers of multikinase inhibitors that are currently undergoing clinical trial assessment and comparison. In particular, a randomized controlled Phase II trial in patients with HCC on second-line therapy showed that tivantinib (ARQ 197), a specific inhibitor of Met oncogene, had increased overall survival in that subset of patients with tumors having high levels of its Met target.

6. An array of newer therapies of different drug classes aimed at a wide range of targets in cell growth, apoptosis, autophagy, and tumor invasion pathways.

7. Newer regional chemotherapy and radiotherapy regimens and delivery systems.

8. The extension of liver transplantation to larger HCCs and its wider availability through use of living-related organ donors; the development of a more flexible liver transplantation patient selection process. For example, the Metroticket model aims to survey patients transplanted outside of the Milan criteria, and to also provide a prognostic calculator to give physicians and their patients an estimated survival prediction after liver transplantation.

9. New radiological techniques to assess the changes in HCC vascularity associated with angiogenic drug actions.

10. Re-evaluation of the use of tumor biopsy to obtain molecular signatures.

11. Recognition of the importance of non-tumor liver parenchyma (microenvironment) for tumor growth control and as a source of prognostic profiling in patients with HCC.

12. The evaluation of kinase and other inhibitors in neo-adjuvant and adjuvant therapy associated with resection, liver transplant, and minimization of transplant waiting list drop-out; identification of use of a vitamin A analog as adjuvant therapy (peretinoin, NIK-333).

13. Re-evaluation of the role or limitation of tumor responses, as kinase inhibitors can enhance survival without HCC size responses.

14. The development of combination therapies to enhance tumor control rates, by either using molecularly targeted drugs that inhibit differing growth pathways, or kinase inhibitors combined with either chemoembolization drugs or radioembolization with ^{90}Yttrium.

15. Realization of the antitumor role of HBV and HCV treatment in patients diagnosed with HCC.

Summary for patients, families, and caregivers

There has been much improvement in the understanding of what causes HCC as well as its underlying biology. This has led to the refinement and development of new prevention, management, and treatment options for patients with the disease. Medical research will continue to advance our knowledge of HCC and enable further treatment choices for patients with this complex disease.

Further reading

1 Carr BI. Some new approaches to the management of hepatocellular carcinoma. *Semin Oncol*. 2012;39:369-373.

2 Kim WR, Gores GJ Recurrent hepatocellular carcinoma: it's the virus! *J Clin Oncol*. 2013;31:3621-3622.

3 Honda M, Yamashita T, Yamashita T, et al. Peretinoin, an acyclic retinoid, improves the hepatic gene signature of chronic hepatitis C following curative therapy of hepatocellular carcinoma. *BMC Cancer*. 2013;13:191.

4 Muto Y, Moriwaki H, Ninomiya M, et al. Prevention of second primary tumors by an acyclic retinoid, polyprenoic acid, in patients with hepatocellular carcinoma. Hepatoma Prevention Study Group. *N Engl J Med*. 1996;13:1561-1567.

5 Mínguez B, Hoshida Y, Villanueva A, et al. Gene-expression signature of vascular invasion in hepatocellular carcinoma. *J Hepatol*. 2011;55:1325-1331.

6 Zhu AX. Molecularly targeted therapy for advanced hepatocellular carcinoma in 2012: current status and future perspectives. *Semin Oncol*. 2012;39:493-502.

7 Kim SM, Leem SH, Chu IS, et al. Sixty-five gene-based risk score classifier predicts overall survival in hepatocellular carcinoma. *Hepatology*. 2012;55:1443-1452.

8 Nault JC, De Reyniès A, Villanueva A, et al. A hepatocellular carcinoma 5-gene score associated with survival of patients after liver resection. *Gastroenterology*. 2013;145:176-187.

9 Hoshida Y, Villanueva A, Kobayashi M, et al. Gene expression in fixed tissues and outcome in hepatocellular carcinoma. *N Engl J Med*. 2008;359:1995-2004.

10 Utsunomiya T, Shimada M, Imura S, Morine Y, Ikemoto T, Mori M. Molecular signatures of noncancerous liver tissue can predict the risk for late recurrence of hepatocellular carcinoma. *J Gastroenterol*. 2010;45:146-152.

Section 6

Addendum

Useful resources		
Alcoholics Anonymous	www.aa.org	1-212-870-3400
Al-Anon Family Groups	www.al-anon.org	1-757-563-1600
American Cancer Society	www.cancer.org	1-800-227-2345
American Liver Foundation	www.liverfoundation.org	1-800-GO-LIVER
American Psychological Oncology Society	www.apos-society.org	1-866-276-7443
American Society of Clinical Oncology	www.cancer.net	1-888-651-3038
Cancer Care	www.cancercare.org	1-800-813-4673
Hepatitis Foundation International	www.hepfi.org	1-800-891-0707
National Coalition for Cancer Survivorship	www.canceradvocacy.org	1-877-622-7937

B. I. Carr, *Understanding Liver Cancer*, DOI: 10.1007/978-1-910315-02-6_6,
© Springer Healthcare 2014

Abbreviations, extended

See below for an extended list of abbreviations used in this text and commonly used in the field.

AASLD   American Association for the Study of Liver Diseases
AFP   alpha-fetoprotein
ALKP   alkaline phosphatase
ALT   alanine transaminase
AST   aspartate aminotransferase
BCLC   Barcelona Clinic Liver Cancer system
CD   cluster of differentiation
CLIP   Cancer of the Liver Italian Program
CP   Child-Pugh cirrhosis score (A, B, or C)
CT   computed tomography scan
DCP   des-gamma carboxy prothrombin
EORTC   European Organisation for Research and Treatment of Cancer
EpCAM   epithelial cell adhesion molecule
FDA   US Food and Drug Administration
FGF   fibroblast growth factor
FGFR   fibroblast growth factor receptor
GGTP   gamma-glutamyl transpeptidase
HAI   hepatic artery infusion
HBV   hepatitis B virus
HCC   hepatocellular carcinoma
HCV   hepatitis C virus
IGF-R   insulin-like growth factor receptor
JIS   Japan Integrated Staging score
LT   liver transplant
MRI   magnetic resonance imaging scan
MWA   microwave ablation
NAFLD   nonalcoholic fatty liver disease
NASH   nonalcoholic steatohepatitis
PD   programmed death
PDGF   platelet-derived growth factor
PDGFR   platelet-derived growth factor receptor
PDL   programmed death ligand
PVT   portal vein thrombosis
RFA   radiofrequency ablation
ROS   reactive oxygen species
SGOT   serum glutamic oxaloacetic transaminase
SGPT   serum glutamic-pyruvic transaminase
SPIO   super-paramagnetic iron oxide particles
TGFα   transforming growth factor alpha
TACE   transarterial chemoembolization
UNOS   United Network for Organ Sharing
UCSF criteria University of California San Francisco criteria
VEGF   vascular endothelial growth factor
VEGFR   vascular endothelial growth factor receptor